James
Pathony

Intra-Operative Neuropathology
for the Non-Neuropathologist

Cynthia T. Welsh
Editor

Intra-Operative Neuropathology for the Non-Neuropathologist

A Case-Based Approach

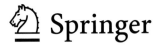 Springer

Editor
Cynthia T. Welsh
Department of Pathology and Laboratory Medicine
Medical University of South Carolina
Charleston, SC 29425, USA
welshct@musc.edu

ISBN 978-1-4419-1166-7   e-ISBN 978-1-4419-1167-4
DOI 10.1007/978-1-4419-1167-4
Springer New York Dordrecht Heidelberg London

Library of Congress Control Number: 2011935368

Printed on acid-free paper

Springer is part of Springer Science+Business Media (www.springer.com)

Preface

Doing neuropathology without all the information you can garner is like crossing some of the less busy city streets without looking first; you can get away with it for awhile, but sooner or later you are going to get hit by a bus. Neuropathologists have extra years of training, but they are also familiar with some secrets that not everyone seems to know.

Neuropathology, much like bone pathology, is much better done in correlation with the radiologic features. There is actually an entire chapter in this book devoted solely to a simplified scheme for differentiating different kinds of lesions based on radiologic features mainly in magnetic resonance imaging (MRI). The differential diagnosis in the central nervous system (CNS) revolves around age and location (information that can also be derived from the scans).

Just because the neurosurgeon sends a specimen for intraoperative consultation does not mean a diagnosis is always necessary to decide what to do next; they probably already have a plan, so relax. If you are not sure of the diagnosis, tell them so. If you can help them with decision making, fantastic! Sometimes you can abort the planned resection of what turns out to be a lymphoma or multiple sclerosis plaque. Also, you almost never need a final diagnosis (just a preliminary), and sometimes the only answer they need is whether they are in the right area, so that ultimately a diagnosis can be derived.

The idea that started the process leading to this book was hatched one day because I wanted to make sure that all of our trainees were familiar with CNS touch preparations and smears. This generally spread out to making this concept available through regional and national meetings by the way of presentations and seminars. When the idea for a book was proposed, it seemed a natural extension. This seems to be a popular theme among neuropathologists currently at courses and finally in book form, which I have been ecstatic to see. Hopefully all of the attention will convince more pathologists, whether in formal training or in the continuing medical education phase, to try intraoperative neurocytology and convince them that correlation with the scans may make the whole process much easier.

Charleston, USA   Cynthia T. Welsh

Contents

Contributors

Zoran Rumboldt, MD Department of Radiology and Radiological Science, Medical University of South Carolina, Charleston, SC, USA
rumbolz@musc.edu

M. Timothy Smith, MD Department of Pathology and Laboratory Medicine, Medical University of South Carolina, Charleston, SC, USA
smithti@musc.edu

Cynthia T. Welsh, MD Department of Pathology and Laboratory Medicine, Medical University of South Carolina, Charleston, SC, USA
welshct@musc.edu

The Role of Clinical-Pathologic Correlation and Use of Cytologic Preparations in Intraoperative Neuropathology Consultation

Cynthia T. Welsh

The after hours call from the operating suite where a neurosurgeon is operating tends to be one that sends blood pressure soaring. It doesn't have to be that way. There are basic steps that can help make the experience much less stressful. Generally you know the age, which narrows the differential considerably. The location, history of the patient (e.g., neurofibromatosis, or known breast cancer), and type and duration of symptoms can all also be very illuminating. We glean the electronic record for information prior to regularly scheduled cases, although that doesn't generally work as well for the evening/weekend emergent surgery. Sometimes, you have to lead your call to the operating room with questions, before you can give any kind of useful answers! It never fails to amaze us how often one piece of clinical information clears up the most confusing issues about which you've been sitting agonizing at the microscope. The radiological characteristics of the lesion can be among the MOST important collection of facts in compiling a differential (e.g., well-circumscribed versus infiltrative, enhancing versus nonenhancing, diffusion and perfusion characteristics and location). This is why there is an entire chapter in this book from a neuroradiologist, in addition to the scans included with each case history presented here.

Intraoperative pathology consultations from the neurosurgeon don't require the same answers that need to be in the final diagnosis. Just knowing the limits of what the neurosurgeon really has to know can make you less anxious. Some questions have intraoperative repercussions, such as with the primary spinal cord tumor; the operation for an ependymoma is quite different from that for an astrocytoma of *any* type or grade. On the other hand, knowing that an adult cerebral tumor is a high grade glioma is often all the neurosurgeon wants to know intraoperatively (not how high a grade or whether there is an oligodendroglial component). The object of inspecting the biopsy, particularly computed tomography (CT)-guided

biopsy, may be simply to assure acquisition of material that will ultimately be diagnostic (not necessarily make the diagnosis intraoperatively). So it may be that all you have to tell them is "yes this is a good area to acquire more tissue for diagnosis." Of course, if you haven't frozen the cores in entirety, then you will have material available that will give you higher quality histology, without risking more core biopsies. Don't assume there will be another specimen; ask. In some cases, the intraoperative consultation can be instrumental in preventing further resection which would be of no use, and could actually be potentially detrimental for the patient, such as if the diagnosis is multiple sclerosis or primary lymphoma. You may be able to suggest microbiology, flow cytometry, or other useful modalities based on what you see. If you have tumor and aren't sure what kind, but can give a differential and/or idea of what grade or how aggressive you believe it to be, just that information may be helpful to the neurosurgeon. But remember, even though it is brain, asking for more tissue is often an option if you are struggling with knowing what the lesion may be (many tumors are huge!). Telling the neurosurgeon you think he is close to something, but not directly in a diagnostic area, is also permissible (and may lead him in the right direction).

Legitimate questions at intraoperative consultation (because they affect the surgery):
1. Diagnostic tissue present?
2. Neoplastic versus non-neoplastic?
3. Metastasis versus primary?
4. Glial versus lymphoma?
5. Low grade versus high grade?
6. Ependymal versus other glial?
7. Recurrent tumor versus radiation necrosis?

Frozen sections in neuropathology have some distinct problems (Table 1.1). There is more of a tendency toward ice crystal artifact than in almost any other intraoperative frozen section, because of the normally higher water content in the central nervous system (CNS). When you add in a lesion (and edema) then the ice crystals can make the tissue unrecognizable as brain, much less diagnostic (Fig. 1.1a). Ice crystals are also unfortunate because of the similarity to

C.T. Welsh (✉)
Department of Pathology and Laboratory Medicine,
Medical University of South Carolina, Charleston, SC 29425, USA
e-mail: welshct@musc.edu

C.T. Welsh (ed.), *Intra-Operative Neuropathology for the Non-Neuropathologist: A Case-Based Approach*,
DOI 10.1007/978-1-4419-1167-4_1, © Springer Science+Business Media, LLC 2012

Table 1.1 Technique

	Cytology	Frozen
Advantages	Better nuclear detail	Architecture
	Quick preparation	Faster scanning than smear
	Miniscule sample size required	Astrocyte processes may stand out
	Easier to recognize macrophages	
	Astrocyte processes stand out	
Disadvantages	Experience helps	Experience helps
	Time intensive interpretation	Wrinkling and folding over
	Assessing cellularity	No "haloes"
	Assessing infiltration	Effacement of vessels
		Effacement of macrophages
		Degranulation of pituicytes
		"Ice crystal" artifact
		Nuclear changes

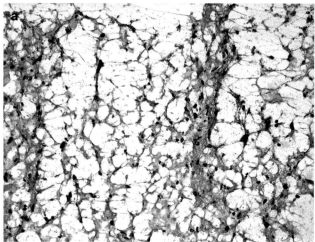
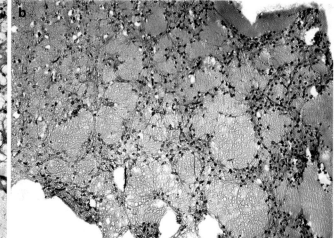

Fig. 1.1 (**a**) Ice crystal artifact. The water content of normal brain is high, lesions make it even higher. The attendant frozen artifact can sometimes make it impossible to tell what type of tissue it is, much less what the problem is. The spaces tend to be angular (more like fissures or cracks than microcysts). Freezing the tissue more quickly, such as with liquid nitrogen or isopentane may help, and a cytology preparation is also useful. (**b**) Microcysts. Microcysts tend to be less angular and have smoother walls. If the tissue is well stained, then the fluid within the cysts will be apparent also

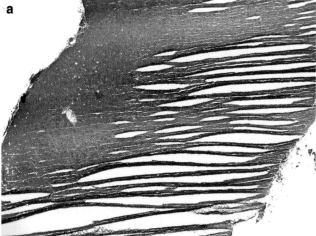
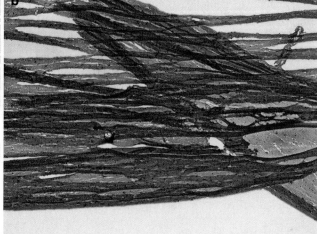

Fig. 1.2 (**a**, **b**) Frozen section tearing and folding. All frozen sections are inherently prone to operator and equipment issues. CNS tissue is really no different and the same management issues apply, such as temperature, section thickness, and blade sharpness

one of the diagnostic features of some brain tumors, namely microcysts (Fig. 1.1b). Ice crystal artifact can be overcome to some extent by freezing the tissue more quickly (e.g., in liquid nitrogen or isopentane slush). The other difficulties involved include those common to all tissues such as issues with cutting the sections (Fig. 1.2a, b), and nuclear and cytoplasmic changes which unfortunately continue on to some extent from the frozen tissue into the permanent sections (Fig. 1.3a), and the parsimonious amount of tissue often provided by neurosurgeons (even if the lesion is 6 cm!). Tissue from the same tumor, which was never frozen, shows there really is no comparison in detail (Fig. 1.3b). Some of the

problems inherent to frozen sections can be compensated for by cytologic preparations. Mitoses can be seen on cytologic preparations (Fig. 1.4a) where there hasn't been too much pressure applied (which can pull them apart), whereas the nuclear changes in frozen sections can make it difficult to distinguish mitoses from just angular irregular nuclei (Fig. 1.4b). A smear preparation takes very little tissue, just a pinpoint fragment, so it isn't really taking away from the frozen diagnosis; or if you don't want to use even that much, you can just do touch preparations, which use basically no tissue. Never forget that it may not be representative if you don't sample all the different areas. Nuclear detail and

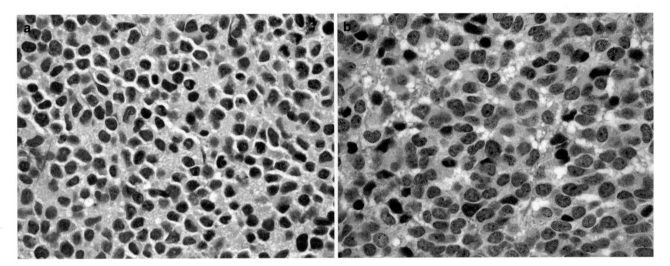

Fig. 1.3 (**a**) Nuclear changes on frozen section permanent control. Nuclei when frozen become hyperchromatic and angular; they stay that way after thawing. This can mislead you as to cell type, if you don't have cytology or tissue that was never frozen. (**b**) Section of the same

tumor that was never frozen. The difference in the nuclear detail between the tissue that was frozen and then thawed (Fig. 1.3a), with the tissue from the same tumor that was never frozen is incredible

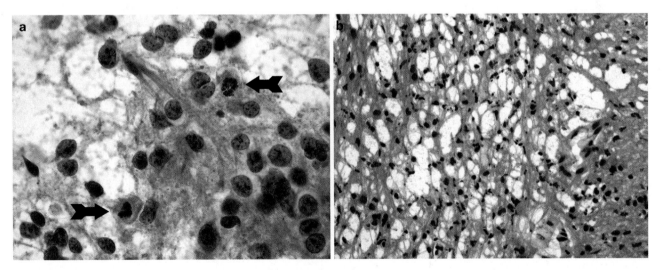

Fig. 1.4 (**a**) Mitoses and nuclear detail on cytology. If too much pressure is applied to a smear, then nuclei, cytoplasm, and mitoses may be smeared also. But with practice, all that detail is going to be beautifully spread out in front of you, and mitoses can be easily found (*arrows*).

(**b**) Angular nuclei on frozen section. Mitoses may be seen on frozen sections, but often are difficult to differentiate from the nuclear changes that freezing causes. Nuclei which were round, may not appear to be so when frozen (and unfortunately remain irregular in permanent sections)

nucleoli are actually useful in a cytologic preparation as compared to most frozen sections (Fig. 1.4a, b). Astrocyte processes are easily visualized on smears, and it is possible to distinguish processes, which are probably normal or reactive (Fig. 1.5) from tumor processes. Some cell types, which tend to blend into the background and can actually save you from making the wrong diagnosis, such as macrophages (Fig. 1.6a), can be seen much better in cytologic preparations. Whenever you see more than a few macrophages or neutrophils (Fig. 1.6b), you have to seriously consider non-neoplastic

conditions in the differential, as most primary tumors have few of either cell type even when very necrotic (unless there has been previous surgery or radiation). Blood vessels are structures that can often blend into the background on a frozen section, such as are seen in hemangioblastomas (Fig. 1.7); these vessels (all vessels really) are easy to identify on smears (Fig. 1.8). The larger the vessels are, the more likely they are to be carried all the way to the end of the slide, along with other structures that don't smear well.

We rarely exclusively crush (squash) the tissue. (Table 1.2) we almost always also smear it to gain thinner layers of cells to analyze. The way the tissue smears allows you to begin making some decisions about it (Fig. 1.9). Normal brain/cord smears very easily and evenly. There are a lot of things both neoplastic and non-neoplastic which smear partly and therefore do not add much information that way. Some tumors (i.e., schwannomas and many meningiomas) and normal structures (i.e., dura) do not really smear at all. These specimens may be more interpretable in touch preparations. If the specimen won't squash easily, you might as well stop at that point instead of adding artifact, because it won't smear well either. You may want to pull the tissue off the slide and stain the slide at that point as a touch preparation. That large cluster of cells will wash off the slide during staining or keep the coverslip from attaching well to the slide, and may interfere with getting a good look at the other cells on the slide. The squashed clump can be saved for permanent sections. We all know that some cell types such as lymphomas and small cell tumors have fragile nuclei, and may smear too easily (Fig. 1.10a). If you can tell from the history or the

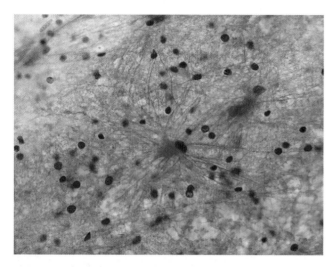

Fig. 1.5 Reactive astrocyte on H&E stained smear. Long, thin processes radiating out from all around the cell suggest it is non-neoplastic; being binucleate suggests it is reactive

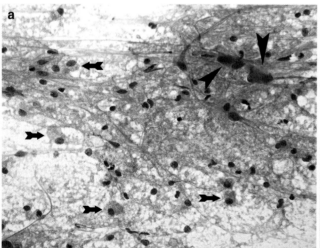
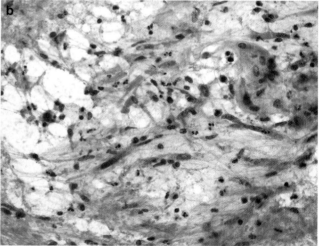
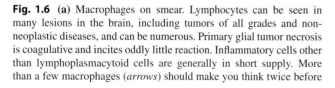

Fig. 1.6 (a) Macrophages on smear. Lymphocytes can be seen in many lesions in the brain, including tumors of all grades and non-neoplastic diseases, and can be numerous. Primary glial tumor necrosis is coagulative and incites oddly little reaction. Inflammatory cells other than lymphoplasmacytoid cells are generally in short supply. More than a few macrophages (arrows) should make you think twice before calling something a tumor that has had no treatment. After surgery, or radiation therapy, macrophages may be numerous. The astrocytes (arrowheads) appear reactive. (b) Neutrophils on smear. Primary glial coagulative necrosis does not usually incite a neutrophil response either, so you should seriously consider non-neoplastic diagnoses in this case also

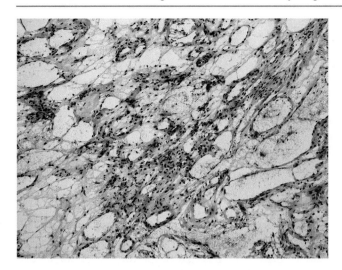

Fig. 1.7 Frozen section of hemangioblastoma. Vessels, microcysts, and ice crystal artifact may blend together in frozen sections. This frozen section could be mistaken for a number of other types of tumors

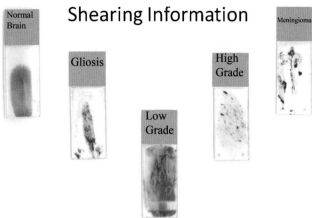

Fig. 1.9 Comparison of tissue smearing. The way the tissue smears (or doesn't smear) can be the next piece of information you collect after the clinico-radiologic information. Normal tissue smears evenly. Gliosis and low grade glial tumors tend to clump (often around vessels). Meningiomas vary and schwannomas generally will not smear at all

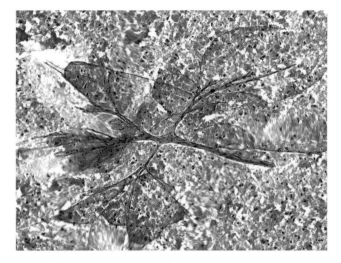

Fig. 1.8 Smear of normal blood vessel. Normal vessel caliber decreases as the vessels branch

Table 1.2 Specimen

	Recommended cytologic preparation	Recommended stain
Pituitary	Touch	
Lymphoma	Touch	Diff-Quik
Uncrushable	Touch	H&E
Most other	Smear	H&E

scans that these diagnoses are under consideration, you can apply more appropriate levels of pressure on your smears or make touch preparations instead. Or if the artifact occurs (for whatever reason) going back and getting touch preparations could be helpful (Fig. 1.10b). Of course, this only works if you didn't freeze the entire remaining specimen.

It is often a good choice to freeze only part of the specimen if it is possible, because of the tissue loss involved and the other losses of information that can be at least partially irretrievable (Fig. 1.3). Smearing of cytoplasm also happens and applying too much pressure can make it appear that processes are present on cells that don't normally have them (Fig. 1.11). Notice the cytoplasmic streaming is all on ONE direction, the direction of the pull, helping you recognize it as artifact. Smearing (and tearing) of the delicate cytoskeleton that holds the oligodendroglial cytoplasm together is what often makes these nuclei "naked" in smears.

One specimen type that we routinely perform touch preparations on, instead of smears, is pituitary. The rationale is that, in addition to the cytology detail, a touch preparation also gives you a sense of the reticulin network holding the tissue together. This network is very intricate in normal anterior pituitary, very few cells other than red blood cells (RBCs) will be present on the slide (Fig. 1.12a), and reticulin is negligible in pituitary adenomas giving you nice cell buttons (Fig. 1.12b). Just remember to make many touches over the length of the slide to clear the RBCs off the outside of the specimen, then you can get an idea how many epithelial cells are coming off the tissue.

Without constant filtering of your stains (whether H&E or whatever else) debris can be a confounder when looking for the coagulative necrosis to which brain is prone; although, sometimes it is fairly easy to distinguish stain precipitant and RBCs (Fig. 1.13a) from tumor necrosis (Fig. 1.13b).

Start by deciding which stain you are comfortable with using on cytologic preparations (Table 1.3). If you like Diff-Quik stains for your other cytology, they are an alternative for this purpose also (whether air dried or fixed Diff-Quik). If you prefer H&E stains, then air drying can be a big

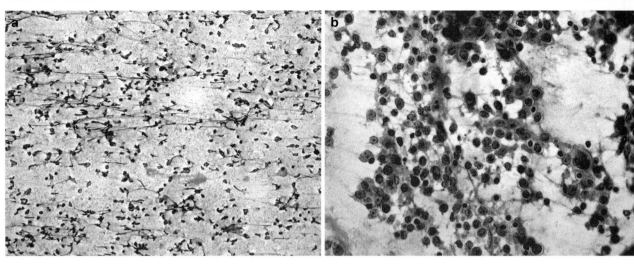

Fig. 1.10 (**a**) Smearing of fragile nuclei. The nuclear fragility characteristically seen in tissue sections of lymphomas and small cell carcinomas in particular is also an issue in smears. Knowing that the patient has a small cell lung tumor, systemic lymphoma, or a primary brain tumor closer to the ventricles than centrally white matter based (which makes you think PCNSL) may make touch preparations a better cytology specimen. (**b**) Touch preparation showing nuclear detail. Going back and doing touch preparations is possible if you didn't freeze all the tissue

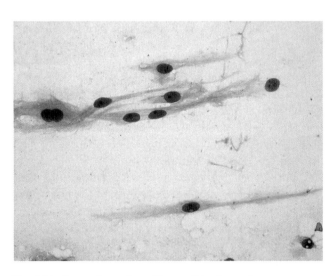

Fig. 1.11 Smeared cytoplasm. If you pull hard enough on smears, you can tear not just nuclei, but even cytoplasm. This can give the false impression of processes, suggesting glial cells, until you notice they all extend in the direction of the pull

problem (Fig. 1.14) and can render them fairly useless, so the slides need to go into fixative immediately. We have our residents fix the smeared slides while they cut the frozen sections, and then run them all through the H&E stain together (saving time and effort). We intentionally use Diff-Quik stains for possible lymphomas of course, they work well for metastases, and often the Diff-Quik stain is what the resident chooses because they want to become more familiar with it. However, we much prefer H&E (Fig. 1.15) Fifstains for almost all specimens. One of the very helpful features on cytologic preparations is determining whether

you have processes on the cells (making them astrocytes) and whether the processes are many/fine (reactive) or few/short/fat (tumor), is something best seen on H&E stains (Fig. 1.5). Just remember to have the fixative right in front of you (not on the other side of the room) when you pull the two smears apart (Fig. 1.16).

We are very pattern (architecture) oriented and like to see a frozen section as well as the cytology preparation, which we feel are complimentary. We almost never rely only on smears, but some institutions do. We feel cellularity is information that is only reliably obtained from frozen sections at our institution, not cytology, perhaps because we have so many different people (with many levels of training) doing the preparations. There can be occasions where due to technical difficulties with the cytology preparations, the only answer may be on the frozen section slide (if it is a schwannoma you aren't going to get a cytologic preparation). Abnormal astrocyte cytoplasm actually often shows up very well on frozen sections (Fig. 1.17), whether reactive or low grade neoplasm, at least in part due to the edematous background. You can get some idea about the morphology of the processes (although not as well as on the smears), and you can see the spacing of the cells (information not available from the smears). Reactive astrocytes cause only just so much cellularity, do not become back to back, and tend not to cluster a lot. They often become binucleate, and their processes progressively become more peculiar, sometimes approaching the changes seen in tumor processes (fewer, shorter, and/or stumpier). It is often a good choice to freeze only part of the specimen if it is possible, but you have to weigh this choice against the

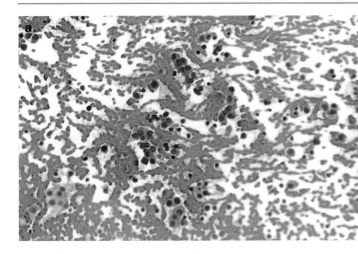
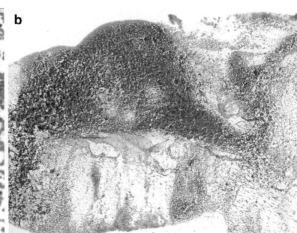

Fig. 1.12 (**a**) Touch preparation of normal anterior pituitary. There is such a complex reticulin network holding the anterior pituitary nests together that very few cells will come off on just a touch preparation. (**b**) Touch preparation of pituitary adenoma. If you smear as little as possible, then you know the cells you are looking at are NOT normal anterior pituitary. Of course, you will have to get closer to them to determine whether they are actually pituitary adenoma, or something else

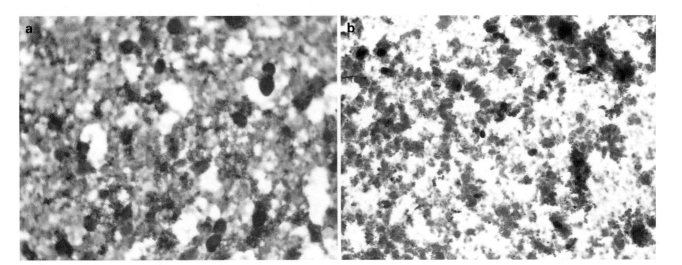

Fig. 1.13 (**a**) Stain precipitant and RBCs on smear. Stains need frequent filtering to prevent artifactual debris being confused with actual tissue debris from necrosis. (**b**) Necrotic melanoma on smear

Table 1.3 Staining cytopreparations

	H&E stain	Diff-Quik stain
Advantages	Familiarity	Familiar to some
	Stained with frozen sections	
	Cell processes show well	
	Nuclear detail excellent	
Disadvantages	Necrosis interpretation	Separate staining procedure
	Air drying artifact	Interpretation of cell processes
		Loss of nuclear detail

additional time required to go back and freeze the rest, when the first frozens don't give you a clear idea of whether the tissue will be diagnostic on permanent sections, much less give you a frozen diagnosis.

Many foreign materials may be seen in CNS specimens. Surgical materials such as hemostatic agents may be present, as well as embolic material introduced prior to surgery (Fig. 1.18). Calcified material can be seen in both frozen sections and smears. Sometimes it is diagnostic material such as microcalcifications (Fig. 1.19a) seen in a number of neoplasms and in some reactive situations, or psammoma bodies (Fig. 1.19b) seen in some meningiomas and some

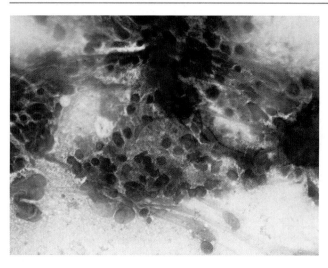

Fig. 1.14 Air drying artifact on smear. Slides for H&E stains must be fixed immediately. Don't pull those slides apart unless you have the fixative right in front of you!

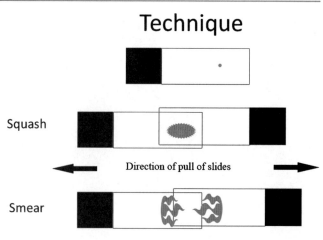

Fig. 1.16 Diagram of squash or smear preparation. You can touch, squash, or squash then smear. Then, either fix or airdry, and use your stain of choice

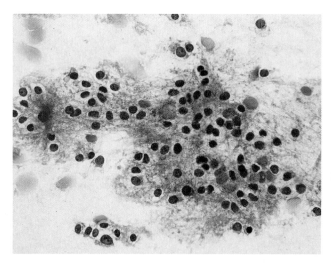

Fig. 1.15 Glial smears. Glial cells have characteristic cytoplasm. Oligodendroglial nuclei generally have a no cytoplasm or a tiny eccentric ellipse of cytoplasm attached. Astrocytes and ependymal cells have more or less elaborate processes depending on cell subtype, which helps you differentiate them from other types of cells. These are visualized best on H&E stained smears, and often also stand out well on frozen sections (Fig. 1.17)

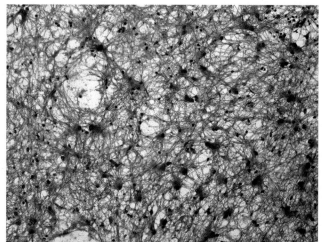

Fig. 1.17 Frozen section astrocyte processes. The beneficial affect of frozen section edema ice crystal artifact on visualizing astrocyte processes

pituitary adenomas, and occasionally they are just corpora amylacea (Fig. 1.19c), but many times it is just bone dust (Fig. 1.19d) from traversing the skull.

Evaluating neuropathology slides intraoperatively starts where you always start:

1. Is this nervous system tissue?
2. If yes, where?
3. If no, what kind of tissue is it?
4. Is it abnormal? Too cellular?
5. What kind of cells are present; are they normal constituents, inflammatory cells, etc.?
6. If the hypercellularity is inflammation and astrocytes, is this reactive?
7. If not reactive, is it neoplastic, and what cells are neoplastic?

To know whether the tissue you are looking at under the microscope is abnormal or not, one of the first things you have to decide is if it is too cellular. It would seem logical, given the variation in cell types and density from one area of the CNS to another, that you need to know the location of the biopsy in the CNS, in order to know what normal should look like. Many times the first intraoperative specimens are not actually from the lesion at all, but are from the surface tissue (often cerebral cortex) that lies between the neurosurgeon and his target. It helps to know what cerebral

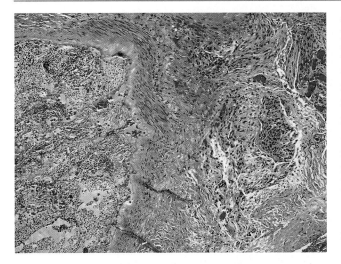

Fig. 1.18 Embolic material in vessel in meningioma. This may make the tissue grossly black. It fortunately for us seldom makes the tissue necrotic enough to be confusing at frozen section

cortex, deep gray matter (Fig. 1.20), and white matter look like on tissue sections and smears to be able to rule out a lesion. Tumor nuclei satelliting around cortical neurons are atypical (Fig. 1.21a) in tumors, in comparison with the normal satelliting of cells around neurons and vessels by normal astrocytes and oligodendroglial cells (Fig. 1.21b), and may be determined to be increased in number also. However, as you can see from the previous photomicrograph of normal temporal lobe (Fig. 1.21b), normal numbers of satelliting cells may be high (this varies from lobe to lobe). Recognizing normal cerebellar cells in smears (Fig. 1.22a) and frozen sections (Fig. 1.22b) is also helpful in distinguishing pathology. Too often internal granular cell neurons are mistaken for lymphocytes (either reactive or neoplastic), or medulloblastoma (Fig. 1.23). Normal vessels in smears can be seen to get smaller after dividing (Fig. 1.8), in comparison to the vessels you will see in high-grade glial neoplasms.

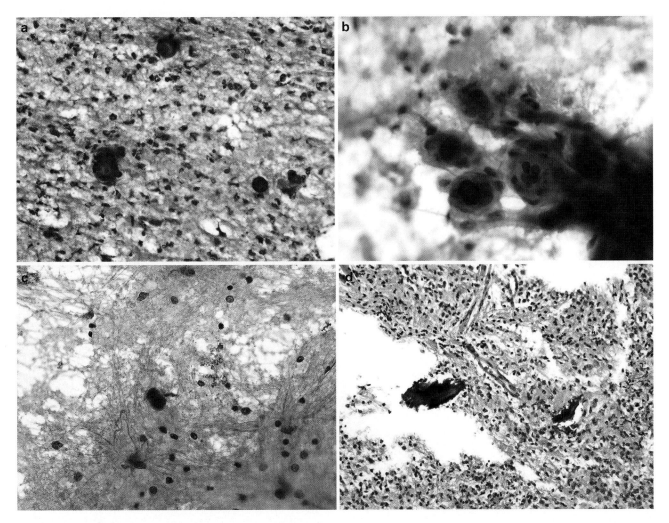

Fig. 1.19 (a) Microcalcifications may be seen in frozen sections and/ or smears. They advance certain diagnoses in the differential diagnosis, so they need to be differentiated from other more common (less helpful) similar structures. (b) Psammoma bodies are seen in meningiomas and some subtypes of pituitary adenomas. They are also present in normal and hyperplastic meninges, so their presence must be interpreted in context. (c) Corpora amylacea increase in number with age and injury (which includes seizures so history can be helpful). (d) Bone dust. Bone dust is common in CNS specimens because the neurosurgeon usually has to go through bone to get there. It is more irregular in size and shape than microcalcifications, psammoma bodies, or corpora amylacea, and tends toward jagged edges

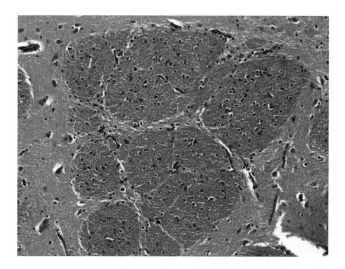

Fig. 1.20 Deep gray matter normally has groups of cells, lacks the neuronal organization of cortex, and has white matter coursing through in bundles. Oligodendroglial cells tend to bunch and line up, particularly along white matter tracts

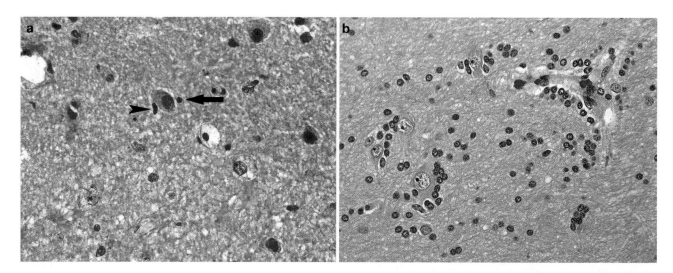

Fig. 1.21 (**a**) Cortex has neuronal organization which can help in recognizing location, and help you tell if there is a lesion. Glial cells satellite around neurons normally (*arrow*), but so do some tumor cells (*arrowhead*). (**b**) Temporal lobe satellitosis. Some areas of cortex nor- mally demonstrate large numbers of satelliting glial cells. Numerous oligodendrocytes line up along vessels. This complicates being able to discuss whether there are increased numbers (which may suggest tumor in the underlying white matter)

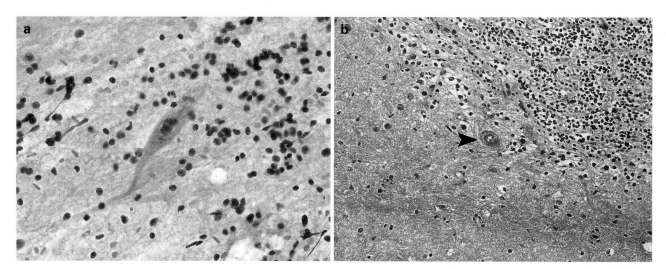

Fig. 1.22 (**a**) Smear of cerebellum. Large Purkinje cells and smaller internal granular cell neurons. (**b**) Frozen section of cerebellum. Large Purkinje cell (*arrowhead*) and smaller internal granular cell neurons

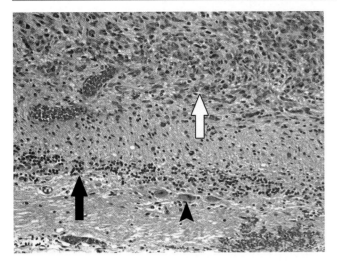

Fig. 1.23 Cerebellum and medulloblastoma. Tumor cells (*black arrow*) contrast with internal granular cells (*white arrow*) and Purkinje cells (*arrowhead*)

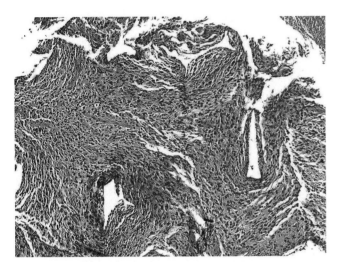

Fig. 1.24 Sponge artifact can distort the tissue to the point where the diagnosis is impaired

When you finish the frozen section, wrap tiny pieces in tissue paper for permanent sections; don't use sponges. Actually, never use sponges on *any* of the soft mucoid type of CNS specimens or you'll end up with a peculiar triangular artifact that distorts the tissue, makes it appear that structures are present that really are not (Fig. 1.24), and can even make diagnosis impossible. Familiarity with the latest tumor classification can be useful at frozen section, although much of the terminology is not something to worry about until working on the final diagnosis (Table 1.4).

Table 1.4 Location-based major tumor differential diagnosis

Skull
Chordoma
Chondrosarcoma
Other primary bone lesions/tumors
Metastases and locally invasive tumors (sinonasal, orbital, head/neck)
Dura/leptomeninges
Meningioma
Metastatic tumor
Meningeal involvement by glioma
Hemangiopericytoma
Brain
Cerebrum
Superficial/cortical-based
Oligodendroglioma
Ganglioglioma
DNET
PXA
Gray–white junction
Metastatic tumor
Subcortical white matter
High grade fibrillary astrocytoma, esp. glioblastoma
Low grade fibrillary astrocytoma
Oligodendroglioma
Hypothalamic/thalamic
Pilocytic astrocytoma
Fibrillary astrocytoma
Periventricular
Primary CNS Lymphoma
SEGA
Septal
Neurocytoma
Intraventricular
Lateral
Ependymoma
3rd
Colloid cyst
Ependymoma
Chordoid glioma
Sellar/parasellar
Pituitary adenoma
Meningioma
Craniopharyngioma
Germ cell tumor
Optic nerve/tract
Pilocytic astrocytoma
Pineal region
Pineal cyst
Pineal parenchymal tumor
Germ cell tumor
Cerebellum
Metastatic tumor

(continued)

Table 1.4 (continued)

Hemangioblastoma
Medulloblastoma
Pilocytic astrocytoma
4th ventricle
Ependymoma
Subependymoma
Choroid plexus tumor
Cerebellopontine angle
Schwannoma
Meningioma
Epidermoid cyst
Brainstem
Pilocytic astrocytoma
Fibrillary astrocytoma
Spine
Vertebral column/extradural
Metastatic tumor
Chordoma (sacral)
Other primary bone lesions/tumors
Intradural (extramedullary)
Metastatic tumor
Meningioma
Cauda equina/conus/filum
Myxopapillary ependymoma
Paraganglioma
Combined intradural/extradural
Schwannoma
Neurofibroma
Cord (intramedullary)
Pilocytic astrocytoma
Fibrillary astrocytoma
Ependymoma

Summary Points (Steps to Achieve the Best Answer Possible for the Patient)

1. Try to get clinical information to know what the differential diagnosis is most likely to be (age, possibly pertinent systemic disease, location of lesion, and radiological characteristics all lead to better stain choices and better differential diagnosis)
2. Sample all sites of the specimen (necrosis, hemorrhage, normal, etc.) for cytologic preparations
3. Use only a minute amount of tissue in aggregate for the smears
4. Crush and smear between two glass slides for most specimens
5. For H&E staining, fixative should be right in front of you before you separate the two slides!
6. If enough tissue remains, try not to freeze it all
7. Correlate clinical, cytologic, and frozen section information – synthesize!

General References

Journal Articles

1. Jaiswal S, Vij M, Jaiswal AK, Behari S. Intraoperative squash cytology of central nervous system lesions: a single center study of 326 cases. Diagn Cytopathol. 2010 Nov 2 (Epub).
2. Varikatt W, Dexter M, Mahajan H, Murali R, Ng T. Usefulness of smears in intra-operative diagnosis of newly described entities of CNS. Neuropathology. 2009;29(6):641–8.
3. Plesec TP, Prayson RA. Frozen section discrepancy in the evaluation of nonneoplastic central nervous system samples. Ann Diagn Pathol. 2009;13(6):359–66.
4. Goel D, Sundaram C, Paul TR, Uppin SG, Prayaga AK, Panigrahi MK, Purohit AK. Intraoperative cytology (squash smear) in neurosurgical practice – pitfalls in diagnosis experience based on 3057 samples from a single institution. Cytopathology. 2007;18(5):300–8.
5. Plesec TP, Prayson RA. Frozen section discrepancy in the evaluation of central nervous system tumors. Arch Pathol Lab Med. 2007;131(10):1532–40.
6. Iqbal M, Shah A, Wani MA, Kirmani A, Ramzan A. Cytopathology of the central nervous system. Part I. Utility of crush smear cytology in intraoperative diagnosis of central nervous system lesions. Acta Cytol. 2006;50(6):608–16.
7. Shukla K, Parikh B, Shukla J, Trivedi P, Shah B. Accuracy of cytologic diagnosis of central nervous system tumours in crush preparation. Indian J Pathol Microbiol. 2006;49(4):483–6.
8. Powell SZ. Intraoperative consultation, cytologic preparations, and frozen section in the central nervous system. Arch Pathol Lab Med. 2005;129(12):1635–52.
9. Yachnis AT. Intraoperative consultation for nervous system lesions. Semin Diagn Pathol. 2002;19(4):192–206.
10. Roessler K, Dietrich W, Kitz K. High diagnostic accuracy of cytologic smears of central nervous system tumors. A 15-year experience based on 4,172 patients. Acta Cytol. 2002;46(4):667–74.
11. Chhieng DC, Elgert P, Cohen JM, Jhala NC, Cangiarella JF. Cytology of primary central nervous system neoplasms in cerebrospinal fluid specimens. Diagn Cytopathol. 2002;26(4):209–12.
12. Walker C, Joyce K, Du Plessis D, MacHell Y, Sibson DR, Broome J. Molecular genetic analysis of archival gliomas using diagnostic smears. Neuropathol Appl Neurobiol. 2000;26(5):441–7.

Books

1. Joseph JT. *Diagnostic neuropathology smears*. Philadelphia: Lippincott Williams & Wilkins; 2007.
2. Burger PC. *Smears and frozen sections in surgical neuropathology*. Baltimore: PB Medical Publishing; 2009.
3. Burger PC, Vogel FS. *Surgical pathology of the nervous system and its coverings*. 4th ed. Oxford: Churchill-Livingstone, 2002.
4. Louis D editor. *WHO classification of tumours of the central nervous system*. Lyon: WHO Press; 2007.

Neuroradiology as a Tool in Neuropathologic Diagnosis of Intracranial Masses

2

Zoran Rumboldt

Introduction

Basics of CT and MRI

This chapter discusses characteristics of intracranial and intraspinal masses on the primary neuroradiological imaging studies – magnetic resonance imaging (MRI) and computerized tomography (CT). First, a very brief description of these imaging techniques – CT uses x-rays, while MRI shows the magnetic properties of tissues, without ionizing radiation. Both of these techniques operate with digital images – during the actual scanning a huge amount of digital data is being acquired, which is then processed by a powerful computer and converted into images on the scanner. MRI is generally the preferred modality, offering higher contrast resolution between tissues and lesions, and an increased amount of information. CT may offer a more reliable visualization of calcifications and better depiction of osseous morphology. Intravenous contrast agents (iodine-based for CT and gadolinium-based for MRI) are frequently used with both modalities.

CT Terminology

The acquired digital data are converted to images in different ways to make them sharper or smoother (by changing the spatial resolution and noise), and these manipulations are known as algorithms (or filters). The best way to evaluate osseous structures is to use a "bone algorithm," which offers the highest spatial resolution (and highest noise, which is however of minimal significance thanks to a very high contrast between the bright white bone and everything else). On the other hand, brain is best visualized with a "soft tissue algorithm," which minimizes noise at the expense of spatial

resolution (pixels are combined to improve image quality, as the images would otherwise be extremely grainy). Both of these sets of images are obtained from the same scan.

The images are then sent to other computers (or printed on film), where they are reviewed by radiologists. While viewing the images, windowing is adjusted to best show the pertinent anatomy and pathology. Windowing is somewhat similar to adjusting contrast and brightness on TV or monitor screens, and certain preset combinations are regularly used: "bone window" is best for images reconstructed with bone algorithm, while "brain window" is generally used for visualization of the intracranial structures (Fig. 2.1a, b). In contrast to MRI, CT scans are in the axial plane only, however, high quality reconstructed images in other planes are readily available with modern scanners.

Lesion description on CT uses the terms density or attenuation; compared to the adjacent normal tissue an abnormality may be darker (hypodense, of lower attenuation) or brighter (hyperdense, of increased attenuation). Isodense lesions are of the same brightness as the surrounding structures.

If intravenous contrast is administered, pre- and postcontrast images need to be compared. Enhancement is increased brightness (density, attenuation) of a normal structure (Fig. 2.1c) or a lesion (Fig. 2.2b) on postcontrast images; a nonenhancing abnormality stays the same.

MRI Terminology

Clinical MR imaging is based on protons in the nuclei of hydrogen atoms. The two main sources of signal are water and "fat" (a collective name for long-chained organic molecules containing fat). MRI studies include a number of different sets of images, known as pulse sequences, requiring a separate acquisition of each sequence. The main magnetic properties of tissues are T1 and T2 and so the basic MR sequences are T1-weighted (T1w) and T2-weighted (T2w). Water (cerebrospinal fluid) is dark on T1w (Fig. 2.3a) and very bright on T2w images (Fig. 2.3b). With additional manipulations either water or fat can be suppressed. Standard

Z. Rumboldt (✉)
Department of Radiology and Radiological Science,
Medical University of South Carolina, Charleston,
SC 29425-3230, USA
e-mail: rumbolz@musc.edu

C.T. Welsh (ed.), *Intra-Operative Neuropathology for the Non-Neuropathologist: A Case-Based Approach*,
DOI 10.1007/978-1-4419-1167-4_2, © Springer Science+Business Media, LLC 2012

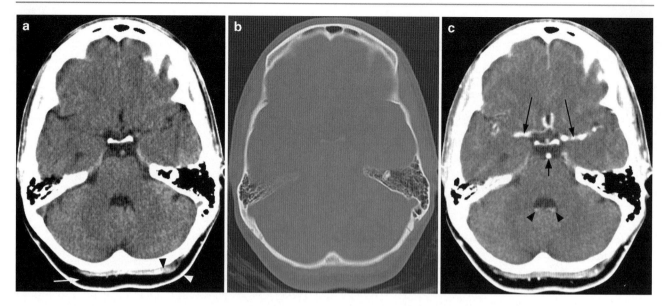

Fig. 2.1 Normal brain CT in the axial plane at the level of the pons. (**a**) Image with soft tissue (brain) filter (algorithm) and brain window, without intravenous contrast (nonenhanced). The bones are white, while the air is black. The CSF is very dark (hypodense), the white matter is brighter, and the gray matter slightly brighter still. The skin and the muscles (*arrowheads*) are brighter (hyperdense) compared to the brain, while the subcutaneous fat (*arrow*) is very dark, approaching the appearance of air. (**b**) Corresponding image with bone filter and bone window. Note that the bones are still very bright, and the air is black, while all the soft tissues are gray with little difference among them. (**c**) Corresponding contrast enhanced CT image with brain filter, the window is slightly wider (less contrast) than in (**a**). Note the enhancement (increased brightness) of the vascular structures – middle cerebral arteries (*long arrows*), basilar artery (*short arrow*), and choroid plexus (*arrowheads*)

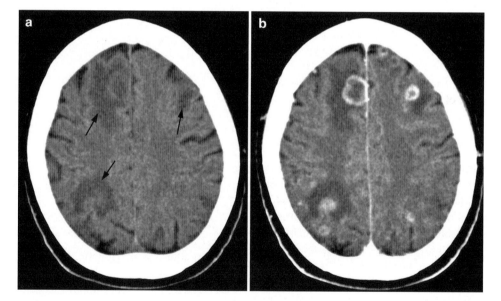

Fig. 2.2 Brain metastases – contrast enhancement. (**a**) Axial nonenhanced brain CT at the level of the centrum semiovale. Multiple bilateral slightly darker (hypodense, of decreased attenuation) areas are limited to the white matter, consistent with vasogenic edema (*arrows* on the larger ones). (**b**) Corresponding postcontrast CT image shows multiple bright enhancing lesions, mostly within the areas of vasogenic edema. Note that the larger masses show peripheral (rim) enhancement

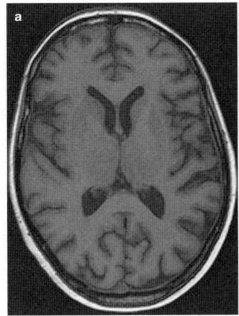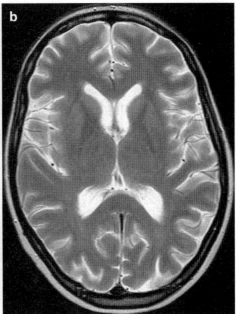

Fig. 2.3 Normal brain MRI in the axial plane at the level of the lateral ventricles and basal ganglia. (**a**) On T1-weighted image (T1WI) the white matter is brighter than the gray matter and the CSF is very dark (hypointense). (**b**) On T2-weighted (T2WI) the white matter is darker than the gray matter, and the CSF is very bright (hyperintense). Very dark lines and dots (*arrows*) are flow voids consistent with vasculature. Fat is bright on both T1WI and T2WI. This is the appearance in adults and children over 2 years of age, the intensity of the gray and white matter is predominantly reversed in neonates and then undergoes continuous changes to reach the adult appearance

brain MRI includes fluid attenuated inversion recovery (FLAIR) images, which is basically a T2w sequence with water suppression (Fig. 2.4a). There are also T2*-weighted images, which are acquired to accentuate artifacts from inhomogeneous magnetic fields, leading to a blooming black out appearance of blood products, calcifications, gas, and metal.

Lesion description terminology is slightly different from CT – brighter is hyperintense (of increased signal), and darker is hypointense (with decreased signal) compared to normal anatomic structures. T1w sequences are also used with intravenous contrast agents. Similar to CT, enhancement is increased brightness on postcontrast images. Frequently used is fat suppression, that eliminates bright signal from fat, for both T2w and postcontrast T1w imaging.

Standard brain MRI also includes diffusion imaging – measuring motion of water molecules. Diffusion-weighted images (DWIs) are a combination of T2-weighting and water diffusion imaging; and water (CSF) is of hypointense signal (Fig. 2.4b). Apparent diffusion coefficient (ADC) maps show water diffusion only and CSF is depicted as very bright (Fig. 2.4c).

MR spectroscopy and MR perfusion are also performed for evaluation of brain masses. These techniques are, however, not widely accepted in routine clinical practice.

Distinguishing Imaging Features

After becoming familiar with the basic terminology, we should proceed to major distinguishing features on neuroimaging studies. Lesion location, primarily intra-axial versus extra-axial is usually clearly evident on imaging studies, resembles gross pathology, and is the first step in evaluation. Helpful signs for extra-axial location are meniscus sign (expansion of the adjacent subarachnoid spaces around the convex mass), inward displacement of subarachnoid vessels (veins), and buckling of the gray–white matter interface. Extra-axial masses commonly also demonstrate a broad dural base (Fig. 2.5), may at times be completely outlined by the CSF, and may cause reactive changes in the adjacent bone. Intra-axial lesions do not expand the subarachnoid space, are surrounded by the brain parenchyma, and may expand the cortex. At times this distinction may be difficult or even impossible, usually when aggressive lesions invade the other compartment (more commonly seen with extra-axial tumors extending into the brain).

The patient's age, while frequently of substantial importance in the differential diagnosis, will not be mentioned in this chapter. Out of many possible imaging characteristics, only the ones that are helpful for discrimination of intracranial masses will be discussed.

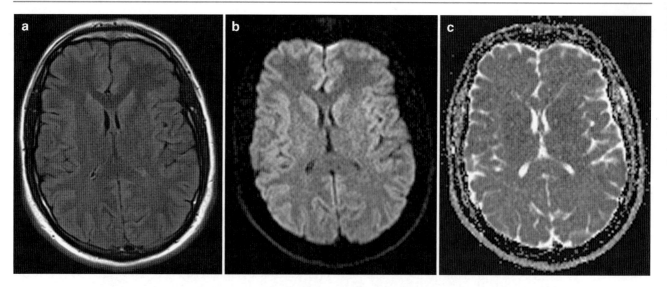

Fig. 2.4 Normal brain MRI in the axial plane at the level of the lateral ventricles and basal ganglia. (**a**) Fluid-attenuated inversion recovery (FLAIR) image shows the white matter as darker than the gray matter, similar to T2WI, while the CSF is very hypointense, as in T1WI. (**b**) Diffusion-weighted image (DWI) is more grainy but otherwise similar to the FLAIR image, however, the fat is not bright. DWI has both T2-weighted and water diffusion properties. (**c**) Apparent diffusion coefficient (ADC) map shows diffusion of water molecules – the higher the diffusion the brighter the signal. Note that the parenchyma is mid gray, with no differentiation between the white and gray matter, typical for brain in adults

Fig. 2.5 Meningioma – extra-axial mass. (**a**) Axial postcontrast brain CT at the level of the lateral ventricles shows a mass (*arrow*) with heterogeneous enhancement, prominent mass effect, and surrounding vasogenic edema (*arrowheads*). On this image the lesion appears to be arising from the right cerebral hemisphere. (**b**) An image at a lower level from the same CT study reveals very bright and homogenous enhancement of the mass, which also exhibits a broad base and sharp margin at the right tentorium (*arrows*), consistent with a dural based extra-axial tumor. Note normal enhancement of the vascular structures

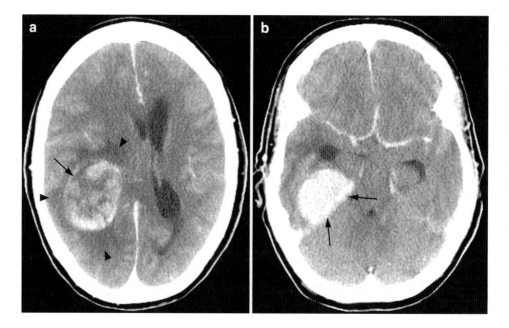

Edema

Many space-occupying disease processes present with edema, seen as darker on CT and T1w MR images and brighter (hyperintense) on T2w and FLAIR images. Two main types can be distinguished: vasogenic and cytotoxic. Vasogenic edema surrounds masses and extends into the white matter, sparing the (cortical) gray matter, and hence having a finger-like appearance (Figs. 2.2 and 2.6). In addition, there is increased diffusion of water molecules in this area, seen as bright signal on ADC maps. In contrast, cytotoxic edema, which is characteristic for infarctions, homogenously involves a well-delineated area including the gray and white matter and extending to the brain surface (Fig. 2.7); the diffusion of water is decreased and infarcts are dark on ADC maps. The term "infiltrative edema" has also been used to describe the pattern frequently present with primary brain tumors – it resembles vasogenic edema, however, the overlying cortical gray matter (and/or the deep gray matter) is also abnormal, at least in some focal areas (Fig. 2.8). Differentiation of edema types is crucial in interpretation of space-occupying lesions.

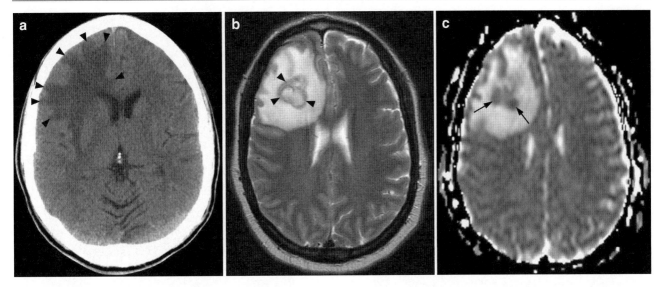

Fig. 2.6 Abscess – vasogenic edema. (**a**) Axial nonenhanced brain CT at the level of the basal ganglia shows prominent right frontal/external capsule vasogenic edema with finger-like hypodense appearance (*arrowheads*) involving exclusively the white matter. (**b**) Axial T2WI in the same patient at a slightly higher level again shows prominent vasogenic edema with bright signal. Within the edema there is a lobulated lesion with relatively dark rim (*arrowheads*). (**c**) ADC map at a similar level as (**b**) shows increased diffusion of water molecules within the edema, while the core of the mass (*arrows*) is dark, consistent with reduced diffusion within tissue debris and white blood cells. Note the preserved cortical gray matter, which is not affected by vasogenic edema

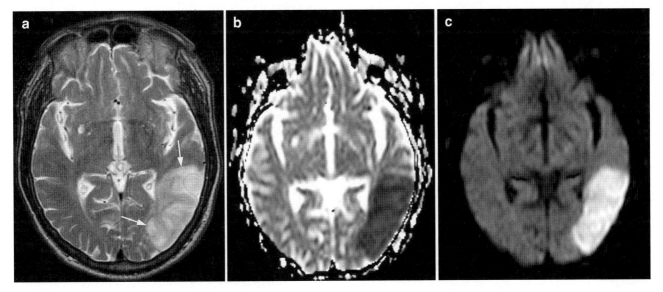

Fig. 2.7 Acute infarct – cytotoxic edema. (**a**) Axial T2WI at the level of the third ventricle and Sylvian fissure shows a well-defined area of hyperintensity (*arrows*) extending to the brain surface in the posterior left temporal lobe that involves both gray and white matter. There is mild associated mass effect with subtle compression on the adjacent lateral ventricle. (**b**) Corresponding ADC map reveals dark signal of the lesion, consistent with reduced diffusion. (**c**) The lesion is very bright on corresponding DWI. It exhibits sharp margins without any finger-like projections

Prominent vasogenic edema (Figs. 2.2 and 2.6):
Metastases
Primary CNS lymphoma (PCNSL)
High-grade gliomas (infiltrative edema)
Abscesses
Granulomas
Toxoplasmosis

Progressive multifocal leukoencephalopathy (PML) (no to minimal mass effect)
Absent to minimal edema (Fig. 2.9):
Dysembryoplastic neuroepithelial tumor (DNET)
Low-grade gliomas
Tumefactive demyelination
Focal cortical dysplasia

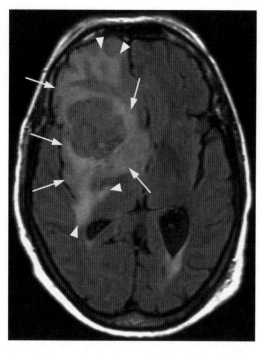

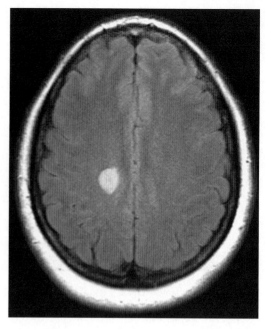

Fig. 2.9 Tumefactive multiple sclerosis (MS) – absence of perifocal edema. Axial FLAIR image at the level of the centrum semiovale demonstrates an oval bright lesion in the posterior frontal white matter of the right cerebral hemisphere. There is no notable mass effect, no adjacent vasogenic edema, and the overlying cortical gray matter appears intact

Fig. 2.8 Glioblastoma (GBM) – infiltrative edema. Axial FLAIR image reveals a lobulated slightly heterogeneous mass in the right cerebral hemisphere, which is surrounded with hyperintense edema. While in some areas the edema has a characteristic finger-like appearance with preserved adjacent gray matter (*arrowheads*), there is also infiltrative edema present with abnormal signal involving the gray matter (*arrows*)

Shape

Lesions may be well-defined with clear margins on imaging, which is true for many benign disease processes (Figs. 2.7 and 2.9), but also occurs with a number of aggressive neoplasms:

Abscesses
Granulomas
Cysticercosis
Tumefactive demyelinationInfarcts
DNET
Low-grade gliomas
Mctastases
PCNSL

Density/Signal Intensity

The disease processes can be further differentiated by their internal structure, most notably by the predominant density (CT) or signal intensity (MRI). A number of masses are characteristically bright on CT and not bright (hypointense to isointense to the brain) on T2w MRI (Figs. 2.10 and 2.11):

PCNSL
Medulloblastoma
All other small blue cell tumors

Granulomas
Adenocarcinoma metastases
Meningioma

Among other causes, hemorrhage within a lesion also leads to a bright appearance on CT and dark on T2w MRI, as is commonly the case with melanoma metastases (Fig. 2.12). A dark appearance is much more prominent on T2*-weighted images, due to signal loss from blood products (caused by their magnetic properties).

Oligodendrogliomas frequently contain even brighter areas corresponding to calcifications on CT (bone-like), which also may be present with cysticercosis, meningiomas, and vascular malformations.

Infarcts are characteristically dark (hypodense) on CT (Fig. 2.13), which is also a feature of pilocytic astrocytomas (including solid portion) and all cystic lesions.

Flow-Voids

Vascular structures known as "flow-voids" are readily visualized on T2w MR images (Fig. 2.14). These are typically present with hemangioblastomas, arterio-venous malformations (AVMs), paragangliomas, hemangiopericytomas, and, in rare cases, with very vascular metastatic tumors.

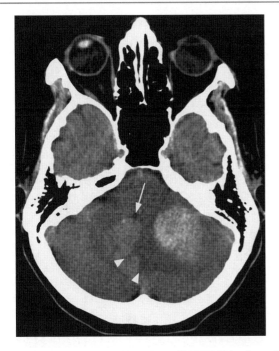

Fig. 2.10 Primary CNS B-cell lymphoma (PCNSBCL) – hyperdense mass. Axial nonenhanced CT image shows an oval bright mass in the left cerebellar hemisphere. There is associated mass effect with displacement of the fourth ventricle (*arrow*) and hypodense vasogenic edema (*arrowheads*). Lymphoma and other small blue cell neoplasms are characteristically hyperdense without contrast administration

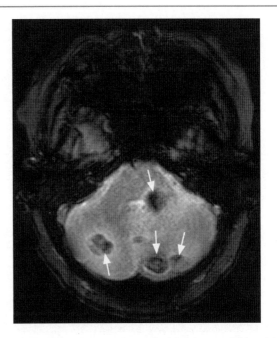

Fig. 2.12 Melanoma metastases – hemorrhage on T2*-weighted images (T2*WI). Multiple lesions with signal loss (*arrows*) are noted on T2*WI axial MR image at the level of the pons, consistent with hemorrhagic masses. T2*WI is prone to artifacts and is visually less appealing than T2WI, however, they are extremely sensitive for blood products, which lead to artifactual signal loss primarily due to magnetic properties of iron-containing hemoglobin

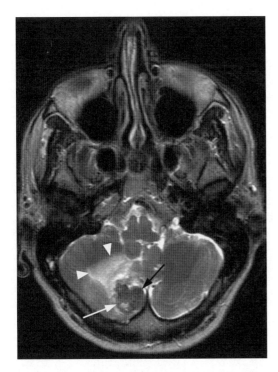

Fig. 2.11 Adenocarcinoma metastasis – low T2 signal mass. Axial T2WI shows a somewhat irregular and heterogeneous right cerebellar mass (*arrows*) that is predominantly darker than the contralateral normal brain parenchyma. Note bright perifocal vasogenic edema (*arrowheads*)

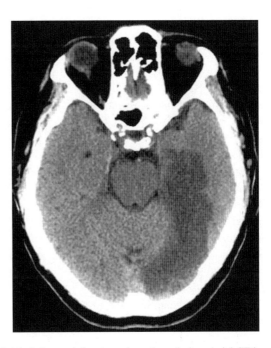

Fig. 2.13 Subacute infarction – hypodense lesion. Axial CT image at the level of the pons reveals a well–delineated large dark area in the left occipital and mesial temporal lobes that extends to the surface of the brain involving both gray and white matter. This is consistent with infarction in the left posterior cerebral artery territory. Compare to the MRI findings of acute infarction in Fig. 2.7

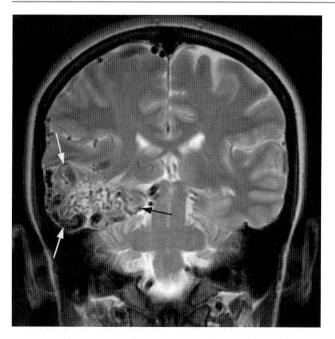

Fig. 2.14 Arterio-venous malformation (AVM) – flow-voids. Coronal T2WI shows a large cluster of linear and punctate flow-voids in the right temporal lobe (*arrows*), with the "bag of worms" appearance, consistent with AVM. Compare to the flow-voids of normal vessels in Fig. 2.3b

Enhancement Patterns

Intracranial masses may or may not enhance with intravenous contrast agents and, when present, different types of contrast enhancement may be observed:

   Nonenhancing (sometimes minimally enhancing):
DNET
PML
Focal cortical dysplasia
Gliomas (even GBM)
   Smooth peripheral enhancement (Fig. 2.15):
Abscesses
Metastases
Cysticercosis
Some granulomas
   Eccentric "target" enhancement (Fig. 2.16):
Toxoplasmosis
   Incomplete ring of enhancement (Fig. 2.17):
Tumefactive demyelination
   Homogenous solid enhancement (Figs. 2.5b and 2.18):
PCNSL (immunocompetent patients)
Some granulomas
Some metastases (without necrosis)
Meningiomas

Diffusion

Diffusion MR imaging is now routinely included in brain MR imaging protocols and low ADC value (dark, hypointense to normal brain) consistent with decreased diffusion of water molecules is a very helpful feature of a number of diverse disease processes (Figs. 2.7c and 2.19). These are listed

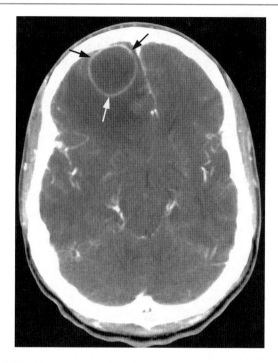

Fig. 2.15 Abscess – smooth peripheral enhancement. Axial contrast-enhanced CT image at the level of the third ventricle and midbrain shows thin and smooth peripheral rounded enhancement (*arrows*) in the right frontal lobe. The central portion of the mass is darker (of lower attenuation). Note also darker perifocal vasogenic edema posterior to the abscess

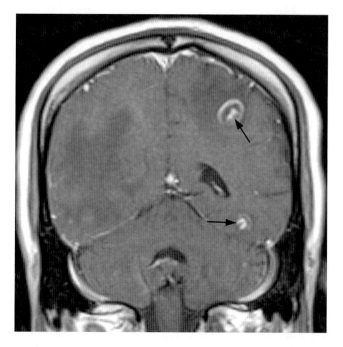

Fig. 2.16 Toxoplasmosis – eccentric "target" enhancement. Coronal postcontrast T1WI demonstrates two enhancing lesions in the left cerebral hemisphere. In addition to the peripheral enhancement of the masses there is also an internal bright area (*arrows*) located off center and adjacent to a portion of the enhancing ring

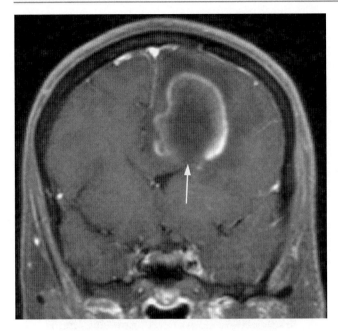

Fig. 2.17 Tumefactive multiple sclerosis – incomplete ring of enhancement. Coronal postcontrast T1WI reveals a large peripherally enhancing mass lesion in the left cerebral hemisphere adjacent to and above the corpus callosum showing mass effect on the ventricular system. The ring of enhancement demonstrates varying thickness and brightness and is completely absent in one area (*arrow*)

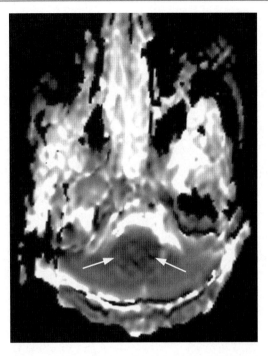

Fig. 2.19 Medulloblastoma – reduced diffusion. ADC map in axial plane through the inferior portion of the posterior fossa shows a dark midline cerebellar mass (*arrows*). Low signal is consistent with decreased diffusion of water molecules within the lesion compared to the normal brain, at least in part due to densely packed cells with very little extracellular space

according to the underlying mechanism responsible for the decreased (restricted) diffusion:

Densely packed cells	PCNSL (solid)
	Medulloblastoma (and other small blue cell tumors)
	High-grade glioma
Pus	Abscess (necrotic core)
Acute inflammation	Tumefactive MS (rim)
	Encephalitis
Cytotoxic edema	Acute infarct

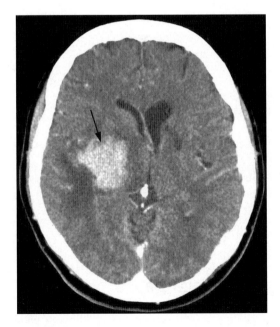

Fig. 2.18 PCNSL – homogenous contrast enhancement. Axial postcontrast CT image at the level of the lateral ventricles shows a homogenous brightly enhancing mass (*arrow*) centered at the right basal ganglia. Hypodense perifocal vasogenic edema is also present

Increased diffusion (bright on ADC maps) is found in a number of tumors, primarily those with a large amount of extracellular space, such as pilocytic astrocytomas (the solid portions), hemangioblastomas, and schwannomas (Fig. 2.20).

Perfusion

Perfusion MR (or CT) imaging is becoming progressively more utilized in evaluation of intracranial masses. Infectious and inflammatory disease processes show decrease in cerebral blood volume (CBV) relative to the normal brain (Fig. 2.21), while metastatic tumors, high-grade gliomas and PCNSL have high CBV (Fig. 2.22); low-grade gliomas

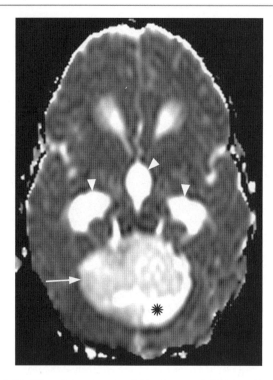

Fig. 2.20 Pilocytic astrocytoma (PA) – increased diffusion. The solid portion of a large midline posterior fossa mass (*arrow*) is very bright on axial ADC map, approaching the appearance of the CSF and cystic portion of the tumor (*asterisk*). This bright signal is consistent with a substantial increase in diffusion of water molecules compared to the normal brain, at least in part due to large extracellular spaces. Also note the dilated supratentorial ventricles (*arrowheads*) consistent with obstructive hydrocephalus

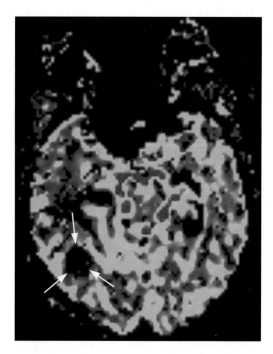

Fig. 2.21 Abscess – decreased perfusion. Cerebral blood volume (CBV) MR image in the axial plane shows a *black* and *blue round area* in the right posterior temporal lobe (*arrows*) reflecting very low perfusion of the lesion

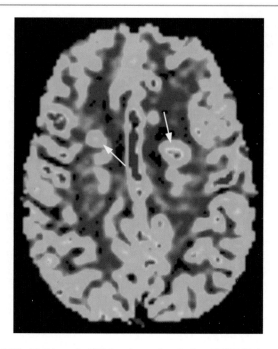

Fig. 2.22 Multicentric GBM – elevated perfusion. CBV MR image in the axial plane shows *yellow* and *red areas* (*arrows*) within bilateral frontal white matter, consistent with very high perfusion of these lesions

generally range from slightly decreased to slightly increased perfusion.

Typical imaging characteristics of individual intracranial masses are listed in the following chapters and illustrated with corresponding figures. The constellation of features is highly indicative for a corresponding lesion; however, there are exceptions to the rule and not every mass will show all the listed characteristics.

Intra-axial Supratentorial Masses

Low-Grade Astrocytoma (Fig. 2.23)

Well delineated, mild mass effect, no edema, centered in white matter – may involve the gray matter, hypodense on CT, bright on T2w and FLAIR MRI, no contrast enhancement, increased diffusion (bright ADC).

Oligodendroglioma (Fig. 2.24)

Involves both gray and white matter, well delineated, mild mass effect, no edema, calcifications common, otherwise hypodense on CT, bright on T2w and FLAIR MRI, contrast enhancement variable, increased diffusion (bright ADC).

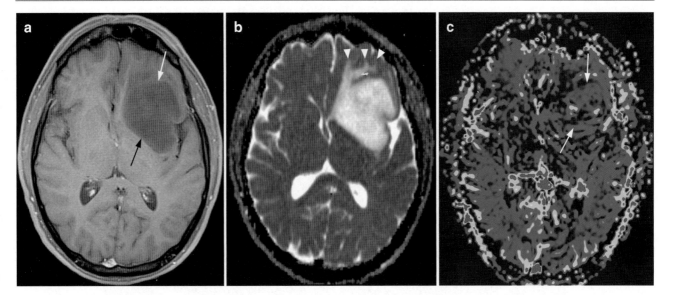

Fig. 2.23 Low–grade astrocytoma. (**a**) Axial postcontrast T1WI shows a nonenhancing hypointense well-delineated mass in the left frontal lobe and insula (*arrows*). (**b**) Axial ADC map at a slightly higher level reveals brightness consistent with very high diffusion within the lesion. Minimal vasogenic edema is noted anteriorly (*arrowheads*). (**c**) Corresponding CBV MR image shows similar perfusion within the tumor (*arrows*) and the contralateral cerebral hemisphere

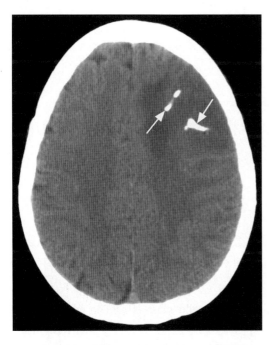

Fig. 2.24 Oligodendroglioma. Axial nonenhanced CT image at the level of centrum semiovale shows a left frontal hypodense mass with internal very hyperdense structures (*arrows*), of similar brightness as the calvarium, consistent with calcifications

High-Grade Glioma/Gbm (Figs. 2.8, 2.25, and 2.26)

Irregular/ill-defined margins, prominent mass effect, infiltrative edema, heterogeneous, multiple lesions possible, predominantly hypodense on CT, bright on T2w and FLAIR MRI, heterogeneous enhancement, areas of decreased diffusion

(dark ADC), high CBV on perfusion imaging [necrotic areas do not enhance, show high diffusion and low CBV].

Ganglioglioma (Fig. 2.27)

Cystic component common, temporal lobe, well delineated, mild mass effect, no edema, calcifications possible, otherwise hypodense on CT, bright on T2w and FLAIR MRI, no contrast enhancement, increased diffusion (bright ADC).

DNET (Fig. 2.28)

Well delineated, minimal mass effect, no edema, involves gray and white matter, characteristic "bubbly" appearance with multiple small cysts, hypodense on CT, bright on T2w and FLAIR MRI, no contrast enhancement, increased diffusion (bright ADC).

Central Neurocytoma (Fig. 2.29)

Multiseptated/polycystic, within lateral ventricles around septum pellucidum.

PCNSBCL (Figs. 2.10, 2.18, and 2.30)

Well delineated, homogenous, within white matter, prominent mass effect and edema, multiple lesions possible, hyperdense

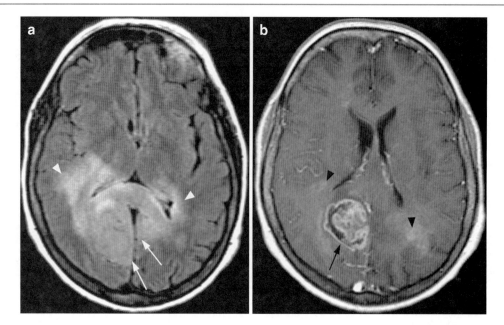

Fig. 2.25 "Butterfly" GBM. (**a**) Axial FLAIR image at the level of the lateral ventricles reveals a lesion centered at the splenium of the corpus callosum involving both cerebral hemispheres. Note the features of infiltrative edema – the margin of the abnormal signal in the white matter is indistinct (*arrowheads*) and the cortical gray matter is involved (*arrows*). (**b**) Postcontrast axial T1WI at a slightly higher level shows heterogeneous enhancement in the central portion of the lesion (*arrow*) and subtle hazy enhancement (*arrowheads*) along the more peripheral areas

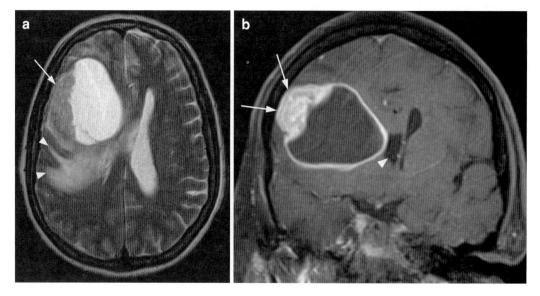

Fig. 2.26 Cystic GBM. (**a**) T2WI in the axial plane shows a large right frontal mass with predominantly very bright internal signal, similar to the CSF, suggestive of fluid. There is finger-like vasogenic edema (*arrowheads*) spreading into the subcortical white matter posterior to the lesion. The lateral portion of the tumor is of different signal, consistent with abnormal solid tissue, involving the white and gray matter (*arrow*), indicative of infiltrative edema. (**b**) Coronal postcontrast T1WI reveals predominantly smooth and thin peripheral contrast enhancement, however, there is much thicker solid enhancement at the lateral aspect of the lesion (*arrows*), corresponding to the solid tissue, which spreads to the brain surface involving the cortical gray matter. Note displaced right lateral ventricle (*arrowhead*)

on CT, not bright on T2w MRI, dense homogenous enhancement, low diffusion (dark ADC), increased CBV [may be necrotic/heterogeneous in immunocompromised patients].

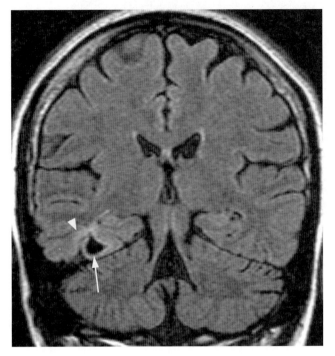

Fig. 2.27 Ganglioglioma. Coronal FLAIR image shows a right temporal well-defined lesion (*arrow*) of central low signal intensity similar to the CSF. There is minimal hyperintensity around this cyst-like mass (*arrowhead*) and no notable mass effect

Metastasis (Figs. 2.2, 2.11, 2.12, and 2.31)

Well delineated, homogenous, or centrally cystic/necrotic, at the cortico-subcortical junction, prominent edema, multiple lesions common, peripheral enhancement (if necrotic) or homogenous enhancement, high diffusion (bright ADC) in the central necrotic portion, increased CBV of the enhancing portion [adenocarcinoma not bright on T2w MRI, hyperdense on CT].

Abscess (Figs. 2.6, 2.15, 2.21, and 2.32)

Well delineated, thin rim of high T1 and low T2 signal, centrally cystic/necrotic, at the cortico-subcortical junction, prominent edema, multiple lesions common, smooth peripheral enhancement, low diffusion (dark ADC) in the central necrotic portion, low CBV.

Infarct (Figs. 2.7 and 2.13)

Well delineated, involves gray and white matter with cytotoxic edema, no vasogenic edema, hypodense on CT, bright on T2w and FLAIR MRI, enhancement possible (usually peripheral "gyriform"), low diffusion (dark ADC), low CBV.

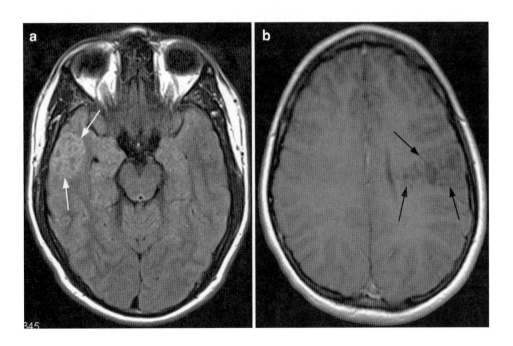

Fig. 2.28 Dysembryoplastic neuroepithelial tumor (DNET). (**a**) Axial FLAIR image at the level of the midbrain shows a right temporal lesion (*arrows*) that is slightly brighter and of heterogeneous "bubbly" appearance. There is no significant mass effect and no surrounding edema. (**b**) Axial nonenhanced T1WI in a different patient again shows the "bubbly" appearance of the left cerebral hemisphere lesion (*arrows*), which extends from the brain surface to the lateral ventricle wall

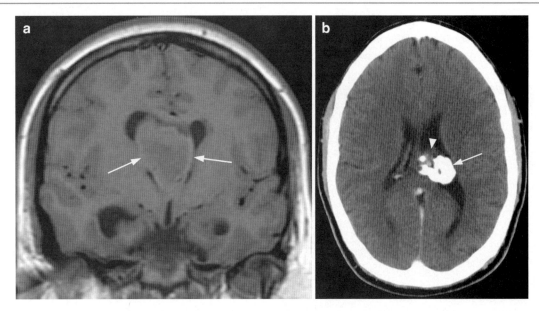

Fig. 2.29 Central neurocytoma. (**a**) Coronal T1WI without contrast shows a midline mass (*arrows*) centered at the septum pellucidum and extending into the lateral ventricles. (**b**) Postcontrast axial CT image in a different patient reveals a mass (*arrow*) extending from the midline into the lateral ventricle. The lesion is predominantly very bright, resembling bone, which is consistent with dense calcifications. There is also a smaller enhancing portion (*arrowhead*) of the tumor

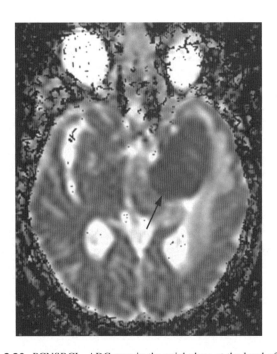

Fig. 2.30 PCNSBCL. ADC map in the axial plane at the level of the Sylvian fissure and orbits demonstrates an oval large dark mass (*arrow*) in the anterior left cerebral hemisphere, consistent with internal low diffusion of water molecules, which is typical for lymphoma and other small blue cell neoplasms. Also note perifocal vasogenic edema with increased diffusion

Tumefactive Demyelinating Lesion (Figs. 2.9, 2.17, and 2.33)

Well delineated, within white matter, minimal edema, multiple lesions possible, hypodense on CT, centrally bright on T2w and FLAIR MRI, peripheral contrast enhancement – "incomplete ring enhancement," centrally high diffusion and peripheral low diffusion, low CBV.

PML (Fig. 2.34)

Prominent vasogenic edema, absent to minimal mass effect, no focal lesion within the edema, absent to minimal contrast enhancement, multiple lesions possible, increased diffusion (bright ADC), low CBV.

Intra-axial Infratentorial Masses

PA (Figs. 2.20 and 2.35)

Well delineated, hypodense on CT, contrast enhancement, high diffusion (bright ADC) of enhancing/solid portion.

Fig. 2.31 Metastasis. (**a**) There are four heterogeneous, round to oval masses (*arrows*) on this axial T2WI image at the level of the lateral ventricles. Most lesions contain large central areas of very high signal (*asterisk*), indicative of fluid and/or necrosis. Prominent vasogenic edema is found around large lesions. (**b**) Corresponding DWI reveals very low signal of the central areas that is similar to the CSF. This is consistent with free motion of water molecules within the necrotic fluid and not to viscous pus

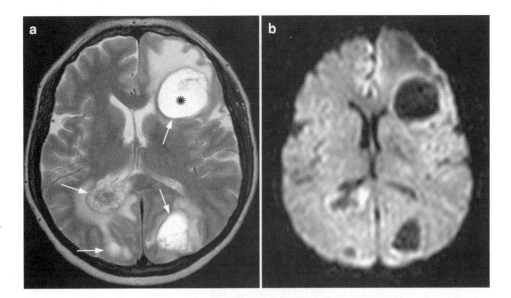

Fig. 2.32 Abscess. (**a**) T2WI in the axial plane at the level of the lateral ventricles shows two masses (*arrows*) in the right cerebral hemisphere. Both lesions exhibit dark rim and central increased signal, similar to Fig. 2.31a. Also note prominent perifocal vasogenic edema. (**b**) On the corresponding DWI image both masses are bright "light bulbs," consistent with a prominent reduction in diffusion of water, as found in dense, viscous pus. Compare to Fig. 2.31b

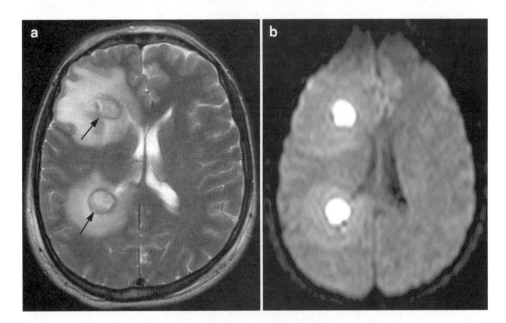

Fig. 2.33 Tumefactive MS. (**a**) Postcontrast T1WI in the axial plane shows a rim enhancing mass (*arrow*) in the right centrum semiovale. The central portion of the lesion is of low signal intensity while the enhancing ring is incomplete and absent in its lateral aspect (*arrowheads*). (**b**) Corresponding DWI also shows peripheral brightness and central low signal. This constellation of findings is characteristic for tumefactive demyelinating lesions

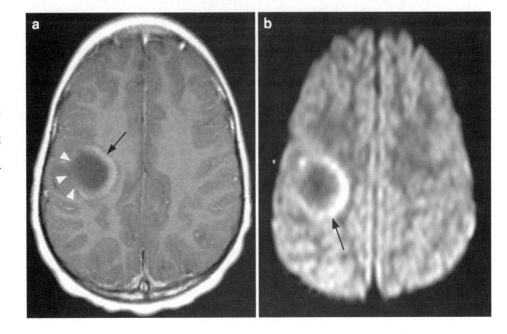

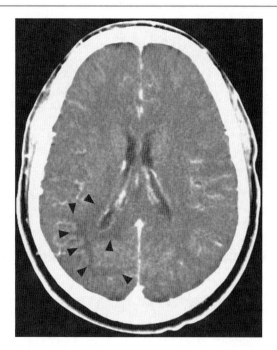

Fig. 2.34 Progressive multifocal leukoencephalopathy (PML). Postcontrast axial CT image at the level of lateral ventricles reveals a darker area within the right posterior cerebral white matter (*arrowheads*) with finger-like projections extending into the subcortical white matter, corresponding to vasogenic edema. There is no associated mass effect or enhancement

Medulloblastoma (Figs. 2.19 and 2.36)

Within fourth ventricle, hyperdense on CT, contrast enhancement, low diffusion (dark ADC).

Ependymoma (Fig. 2.37)

Heterogeneous, calcifications and hemorrhage common, within fourth ventricle, extending through the foramina, contrast enhancement, heterogeneous diffusion.

Hemangioblastoma (Fig. 2.38)

Well delineated, hypodense on CT, prominent flow-voids on T2w MRI, contrast enhancement, high diffusion (bright ADC).

Subependymoma (Fig. 2.39)

Well delineated, within fourth ventricle, absent to minimal enhancement, high diffusion (bright ADC).

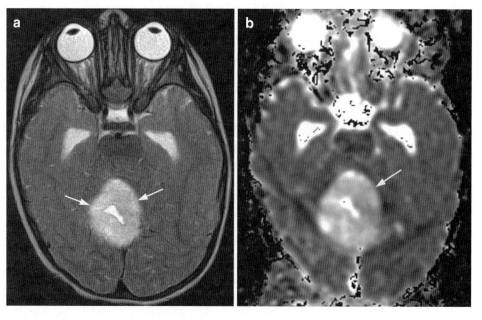

Fig. 2.35 PA. (**a**) Axial T2WI shows a midline infratentorial mass (*arrows*) with increased signal. (**b**) Corresponding ADC map shows that the tumor (*arrow*) is brighter than the brain, consistent with relatively increased diffusion of water molecules

Fig. 2.36 Medulloblastoma. (a) A heterogeneous midline mass (*arrows*) centered at the fourth ventricle is depicted on T2WI in the axial plane. (b) Corresponding ADC map shows that the tumor (*arrow*) is darker than the brain, consistent with relative decrease in diffusion of water. Compare to Fig. 2.35a

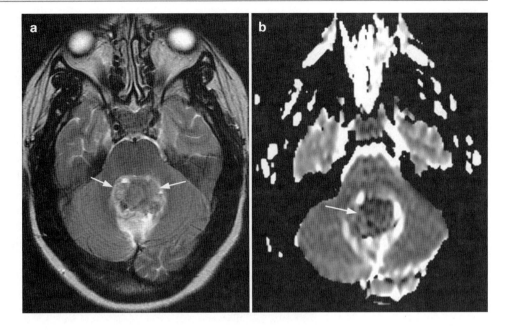

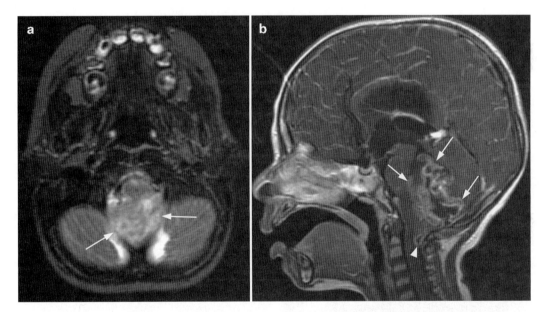

Fig. 2.37 Ependymoma. (a) Axial T2WI at the inferior aspect of the posterior fossa shows a heterogeneous predominantly bright mass (*arrows*) extending through the foramen of Magendie, just posterior to the spinal cord. (b) Midsagittal post contrast T1WI reveals heterogeneous enhancement of the lesion (*arrows*), which fills the fourth ventricle. Inferior extension through the foramen of Magendie is again shown (*arrowhead*)

Metastasis (Figs. 2.11 and 2.31)

Well delineated, homogenous or centrally cystic/necrotic, prominent edema, multiple lesions common, peripheral enhancement (if necrotic) or homogenous enhancement, high diffusion (bright ADC) in the central necrotic portion, increased CBV of the enhancing portion [adenocarcinoma not bright on T2w MRI, hyperdense on CT].

Extra-axial Supra/Infratentorial Masses

Meningioma (Figs. 2.5 and 2.40)

Well delineated, homogenous, "dural tail," hyperdense on CT, not bright on T2w MRI, dense homogenous enhancement, underlying bone not invaded [unless intraosseus meningioma – epicenter within the bone, sphenoid wing].

Fig. 2.38 Hemangioblastoma.
(**a**) Axial postcontrast T1WI
through the posterior fossa shows
a rounded mass with bright
enhancement (*arrow*). (**b**)
Corresponding T2WI reveals
multiple dark linear structures
(*arrowheads*) within the tumor,
consistent with flow-voids from
intratumoral vasculature

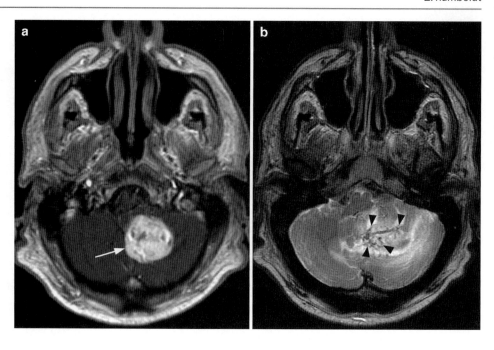

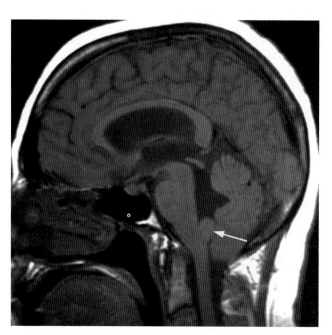

Fig. 2.39 Subependymoma. Midsagittal nonenhanced T1WI demonstrates an oval mass (*arrow*) in the inferior portion of the fourth ventricle, of similar brightness as the brain parenchyma

Systemic Lymphoma (Fig. 2.41)

Well delineated, homogenous, hyperdense on CT, not bright on T2w MRI, dense homogenous enhancement, adjacent bone commonly involved.

Extra-axial Metastasis (Fig. 2.42)

Well delineated, heterogeneous/necrotic or homogenous, primary prostate cancer, contrast enhancement, adjacent bone/scalp commonly involved.

Choroid Plexus Papilloma (Fig. 2.43)

Although choroid plexus papilloma is an intra-axial lesion, on imaging studies it typically appears as an intraventricular extra-axial mass.

Multilobular, heterogeneous, calcifications common on CT, hemorrhage possible, within ventricles, flow-voids present on T2w MRI, contrast enhancement.

Schwannoma (Fig. 2.44)

Well delineated, along the cranial nerves (IAC), homogenous when small, heterogeneous and bright on T2w MRI when large, contrast enhancement, high diffusion (bright ADC).

Extra-axial Sella/Skull Base/Pineal Masses

Pituitary Adenoma (Fig. 2.45)

Intrasellar, suprasellar extension common, enhancement less than the normal pituitary gland, cystic, and hemorrhagic changes possible.

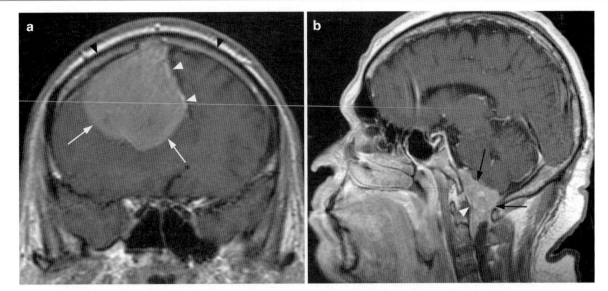

Fig. 2.40 Meningioma. (**a**) Postcontrast T1WI in the coronal plane shows a large homogenously enhancing bright mass (*arrows*). The lesion has a broad base along the falx (*white arrowheads*), which is displaced to the left, consistent with a parafalcine meningioma. Note the normal bright signal of the fatty bone marrow (*black arrowheads*) in the calvarium adjacent to the tumor and on the other side. (**b**) Sagittal postcontrast T1WI in a different patient demonstrates a bright homogenously enhancing mass (*arrows*) with a broad base (*arrowhead*) along the dura at the anterior aspect of the foramen magnum

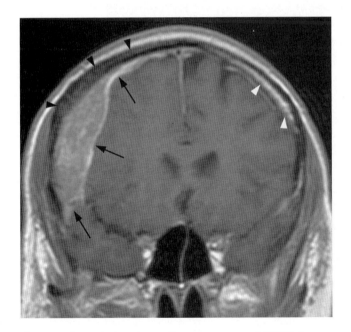

Fig. 2.41 Systemic lymphoma. Postcontrast coronal T1WI shows a homogenously enhancing dural-based mass (*arrows*) in the right cerebral hemisphere. This appearance may be indistinguishable from a meningioma. However, the adjacent bone marrow (*black arrowheads*) has lost its normal bright signal, consistent with infiltration. Note that the contralateral bone marrow has normal brightness (*white arrowheads*). Compare to Fig. 2.40a

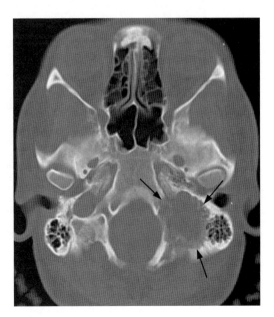

Fig. 2.42 Skull base metastasis. Axial CT image with bone filter and window shows a destructive lesion (*arrows*) at the left skull base. Note the irregular lytic appearance along the lesion margins

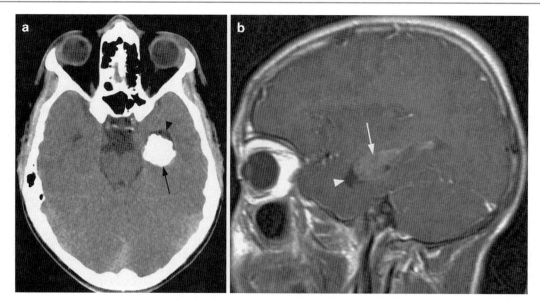

Fig. 2.43 Choroid plexus papilloma. (**a**) Nonenhanced axial CT image at the level of the midbrain shows a very bright mass (*arrow*), similar to bones, within the temporal horn of the left lateral ventricle. Large calcifications as in this case are not common in choroid plexus papillomas.

The tip of the temporal horn (*arrowhead*) is dilated. (**b**) Sagittal postcontrast T1WI through the lesion (*arrow*) demonstrates enhancement of the tumor. Again note the dilated temporal horn tip (*arrowhead*)

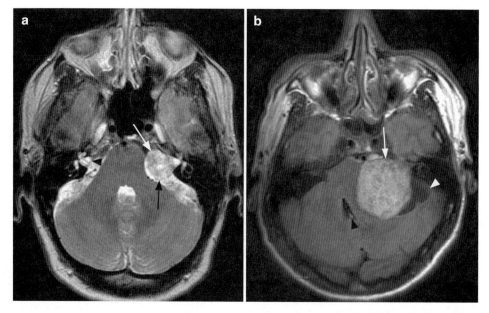

Fig. 2.44 Schwannoma. (**a**) Axial T2WI at the level of the pons shows a heterogeneous predominantly bright mass (*arrows*) at the left cerebello-pontine angle. The internal auditory canal (IAC) is expanded by the tumor – compare to the normal right IAC (*arrowhead*). (**b**) Postcontrast axial FLAIR image in a different patient demonstrates a large heterogeneously enhancing mass (*arrow*) at the left

cerebello-pontine angle. There is trapped CSF (*white arrowhead*) adjacent to the lesion, without peripheral contrast enhancement. Note the prominent mass effect with compression and displacement of the fourth ventricle (*black arrowhead*). FLAIR images may also be acquired (as in this case) following contrast administration, similar to T1WI

Parasellar Meningioma (Fig. 2.46)

Parasellar, commonly centered at cavernous sinus, not bright on T2w MRI, hyperdense on CT, homogenous dense enhancement, dural tail, narrows the internal carotid artery caliber.

Cavernous Sinus Hemangioma (Fig. 2.47)

Parasellar, at cavernous sinus, calcifications possible, otherwise hypodense on CT, very bright on T2w MRI, dense contrast enhancement.

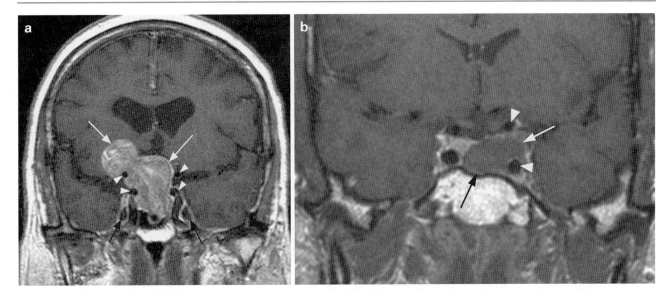

Fig. 2.45 Pituitary adenoma. (**a**) Coronal postcontrast T1WI through the sella shows a large sellar mass with suprasellar extension (*arrows*), especially on the right. The tumor also extends inferiorly into the sphenoid sinus (*asterisk*). The lesion is immediately adjacent to the internal carotid arteries (ICAs, *white arrowheads*). Normal Meckel's caves (*black arrowheads*) are also visualized. (**b**) Coronal postcontrast T1WI through the sella in a different patient reveals a mass (*arrows*) that is centered at the left side of the pituitary gland and shows absent to minimal enhancement. The tumor extends laterally (*white arrow*) past the ICA (*arrowheads*), indicating cavernous sinus invasion

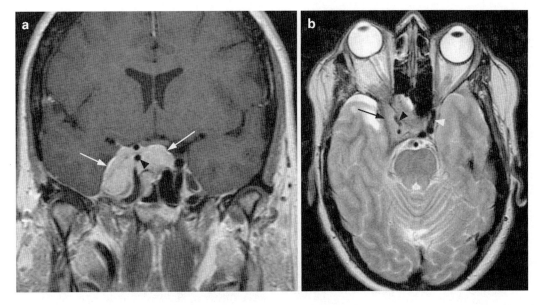

Fig. 2.46 Parasellar meningioma. (**a**) Coronal postcontrast T1WI through the sella shows a homogenous brightly enhancing mass (*arrow*) centered at the right cavernous sinus surrounding the right ICA (*arrowhead*). Note relative decrease in caliber of the right ICA compared to the left ICA. (**b**) Axial T2WI shows homogeneous appearance of the tumor (*arrows*), which is of similar signal as the gray matter and extends posteriorly along the tentorium. Narrowing of the surrounded right ICA (*black arrowhead*) is more conspicuous than in Fig. 2.46a. Normal left ICA (*white arrowhead*) for comparison. In contrast to pituitary adenomas, meningiomas commonly lead to decreased ICA caliber

Parasellar Schwannoma (Fig. 2.48)

Well delineated, along the cranial nerves (Meckel's cave, "dumbbell shape" common), homogenous when small, heterogeneous and bright on T2w MRI when large, hypodense on CT, contrast enhancement.

Craniopharyngioma (Fig. 2.49)

Suprasellar, calcifications very common on CT, (poly)cystic appearance common, otherwise hypodense on CT and bright on T2w MRI, contrast enhancement of cyst walls is sometimes very subtle.

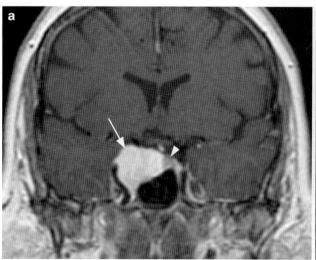 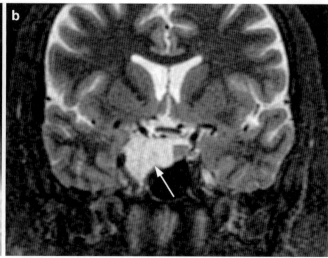

Fig. 2.47 Cavernous sinus hemangioma. (**a**) Coronal postcontrast T1WI through the sella shows a densely enhancing bright mass (*arrow*), which enhances more than the displaced pituitary gland (*arrowhead*). (**b**) Corresponding T2WI image with fat suppression reveals marked brightness of the lesion, approaching the CSF signal – compare to Fig. 2.47b showing much darker meningioma. Also note that the right ICA is displaced but without any narrowing of the lumen

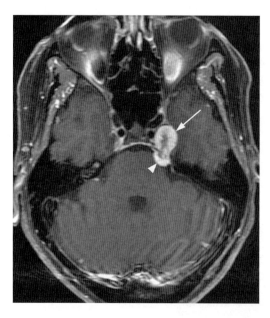

Fig. 2.48 Parasellar schwannoma. Axial postcontrast T1WI with fat saturation shows a heterogeneously enhancing mass extending along the course of the left trigeminal nerve, with one portion lying adjacent to the pons (*arrowhead*) and the other part filling the Meckel's cave (*arrow*)

Plasmacytoma/Multiple Myeloma (Fig. 2.50)

Centered at bone, osteolytic on CT, replacement of normal bright bone marrow on T1w MRI, contrast enhancement.

Chordoma (Fig. 2.51)

At midline, arising from clivus, lobulated, and septated, very bright on T2w MRI, enhancement mild to absent, high diffusion (bright ADC).

Chondrosarcoma (Fig. 2.52)

Off midline (petroclival junction), lobulated and septated, very bright on T2w MRI, calcifications common on CT (chondroid matrix pattern), enhancement mild to absent, high diffusion (bright ADC).

Olfactory Neuroblastoma (Fig. 2.53)

At cribriform plate, sinonasal and intracranial extension, cysts common and characteristic, contrast enhancement, dural metastases possible.

Pineoblastoma (Fig. 2.54)

At pineal gland, not bright on T2w MRI, hyperdense on CT with "exploded" scattered pineal calcifications, contrast enhancement, low diffusion (dark ADC).

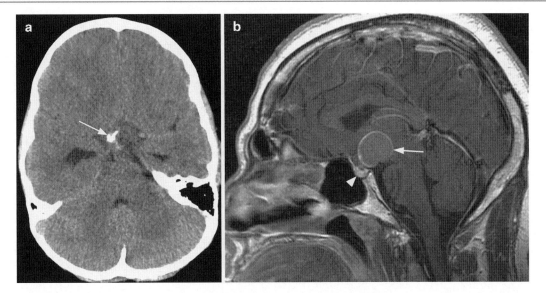

Fig. 2.49 Craniopharyngioma. (**a**) Nonenhanced axial CT image at the level of the suprasellar cisterns shows a very bright right paramedial lesion (*arrow*), consistent with calcification. The vast majority of craniopharyngiomas contain calcifications on CT studies. (**b**) Sagittal postcontrast T1WI shows thin peripheral increased brightness of the rounded mass (*arrow*), consistent with subtle enhancement. The tumor is suprasellar in location; note the normal enhancing pituitary gland (*arrowhead*) within the sella

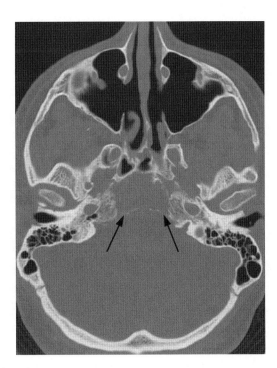

Fig. 2.50 Plasmacytoma/multiple myeloma. Axial CT image with bone algorithm and window shows a destructive lesion of the clivus (*arrows*). Note absence of mass effect and smooth regular margins of the abnormality. Compare to metastasis in Fig. 2.42

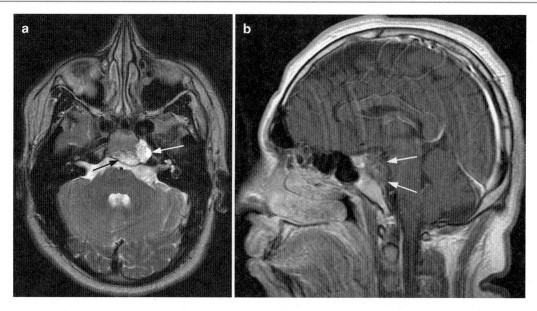

Fig. 2.51 Chordoma. (**a**) T2WI in the axial plane at the level of the clivus and pons shows a bright mass (*arrows*) arising from the clivus at the midline and to the left. (**b**) Sagittal postcontrast T1WI reveals only mild and heterogeneous enhancement of the tumor (*arrows*)

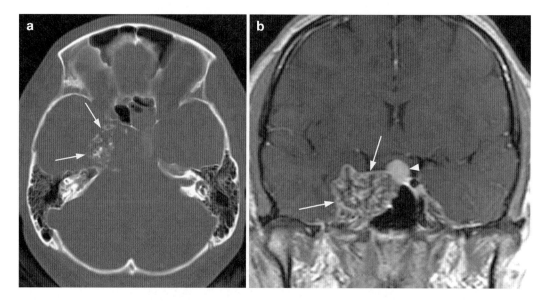

Fig. 2.52 Chondrosarcoma. (**a**) Axial CT image with bone filter and window shows bright coarse calcifications (*arrows*) anterior to and above the right petro-clival junction (*arrowhead*). (**b**) Coronal postcontrast T1WI through the sellar region demonstrates markedly heterogeneous enhancement of the mass (*arrows*) in a linear and punctuate fashion. Note normally enhancing pituitary gland (*arrowhead*)

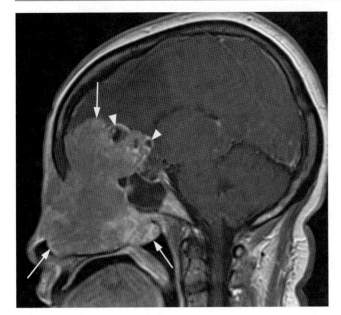

Fig. 2.53 Olfactory neuroblastoma (Esthesioneuroblastoma). Postcontrast T1WI in the sagittal plane reveals a large enhancing mass (*arrows*) with intracranial and extracranial components. The lesion extends from the nasal cavity and nasopharynx to the frontal lobe, with the epicenter and waist at the level of the cribriform plate. The intracranial portion of the tumor contains a few rounded nonenhancing areas (*arrowheads*), consistent with cysts, which are highly suggestive of an olfactory neuroblastoma

Germ Cell Tumor (Fig. 2.55)

At pineal gland, not bright on T2w MRI, hyperdense on CT surrounding preserved pineal calcifications, contrast enhancement, low diffusion (dark ADC).

Spinal Masses

Spinal masses are best differentiated on imaging studies based on their location and patient's age. The primary division is into extramedullary and intramedullary lesions. Schwannomas, meningiomas, and myxopapillary ependymomas are the most common extramedullary neoplasms, while ependymomas, astrocytomas, and hemangioblastomas are located within the spinal cord.

Schwannoma (Fig. 2.56)

Along nerves (neural foramina, cauda equina), oval, well delineated, bright on T2w MRI, contrast enhancement.

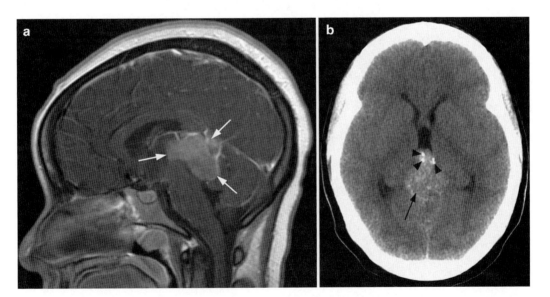

Fig. 2.54 Pineoblastoma. (**a**) Midsagittal T1WI following contrast administration shows a large enhancing mass (*arrows*) in the pineal region. (**b**) Axial nonenhanced CT image through the lesion (*arrow*) reveals its mild hyperdensity. The normal pineal calcifications (*arrowheads*) are separated, "exploded" by the tumor. This is a typical appearance of a pineoblastoma

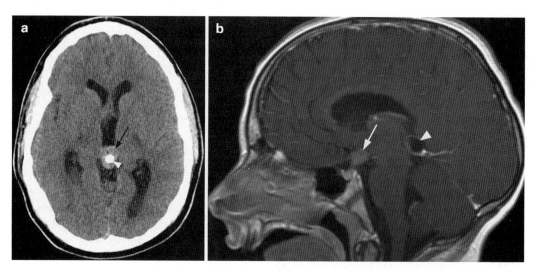

Fig. 2.55 Germ cell tumor. (**a**) Axial nonenhanced CT image at the level of the pineal gland and basal ganglia shows an isodense mass (*arrow*) surrounding intact pineal calcification (*arrowhead*), indicative of a germ cell tumor. Compare to Fig. 2.54b. (**b**) Following treatment the enhancing tumor recurred in the parasellar location (*arrow*), as seen on this sagittal postcontrast T1WI. Note the absence of lesions in the pineal region, which is filled with CSF (*arrowhead*)

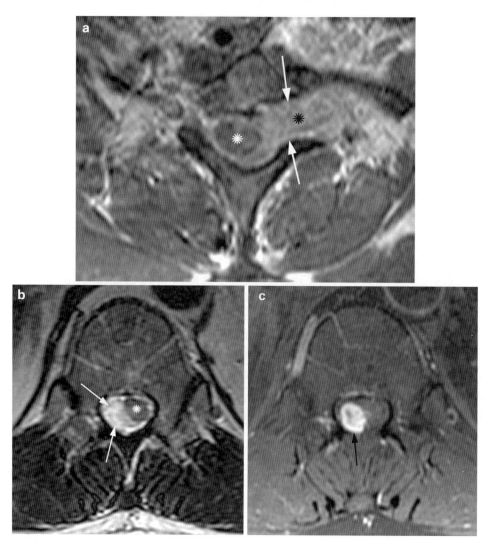

Fig. 2.56 Spinal schwannoma. (**a**) Postcontrast T1WI in the axial plane through the lower cervical spine shows an enhancing mass (*black asterisk*) that is expanding the left neural foramen (*arrows*). The spinal cord (*white asterisk*) is mildly displaced to the right by the tumor. (**b**) Axial T2WI through the lower thoracic spine in a different patient demonstrates a bright mass (*arrows*) within the spinal canal on the right side, which displaces the spinal cord (*asterisk*) to the left. (**c**) Corresponding T1WI with fat saturation reveals bright slightly heterogeneous enhancement of the lesion (*arrow*)

Myxopapillary Ependymoma (Fig. 2.57)

At/adjacent to conus medullaris, lobular when large, bright on T2w MRI, contrast enhancement [when small at cauda equine may not be distinguished from Schwannoma].

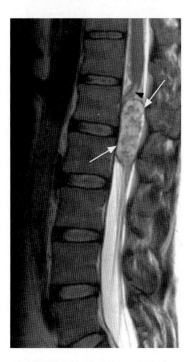

Fig. 2.57 Myxopapillary ependymoma. Sagittal T2WI through the thoraco-lumbar region shows a heterogeneous predominantly bright mass (*arrows*), which is located just inferior to the conus medullaris. There is also a small amount of bright edema (*arrowhead*) within the conus. This is a typical location of myxopapillary ependymoma

Meningioma (Fig. 2.58)

Dural-based, "en plaque" appearance, not bright on T2w MRI, dense homogenous enhancement.

Ependymoma (Fig. 2.59)

Central intramedullary, peritumoral cysts possible, hemorrhage possible, contrast enhancement variable (absent to prominent), occurs in children only with NF-2, multiple lesions common with NF-2.

Astrocytoma (Fig. 2.60)

Eccentric intramedullary, enhancement variable, pediatric population.

Hemangioblastoma (Fig. 2.61)

Along spinal cord surface, contrast enhancement, multiple lesions possible [with VHL].

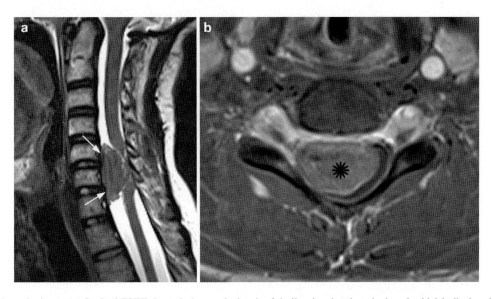

Fig. 2.58 Spinal meningioma. (**a**) Sagittal T2WI through the cervical and upper thoracic spine shows an extramedullary mass with a broad base along the ventral dura (*arrows*) – compare to Fig. 2.40b. The lesion is of similar signal as the spinal cord, which is displaced. (**b**) Postcontrast axial T1WI through the tumor (*asterisk*) shows its homogenous enhancement. The mass occupies most of the spinal canal at this level

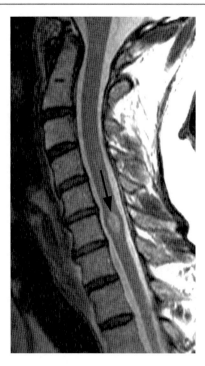

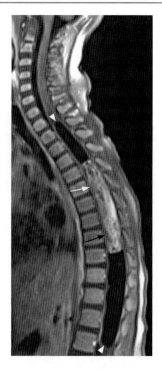

Fig. 2.59 Spinal ependymoma. Sagittal T2WI through the cervical and upper thoracic spine demonstrates an oval bright mass within the central portion of the spinal cord (*arrow*), corresponding to the tumor's origin from the central canal

Fig. 2.60 Spinal astrocytoma. Sagittal post contrast T1WI through the cervical, thoracic and upper lumbar spine shows a large somewhat heterogeneous enhancing intramedullary mass (*arrows*). There are peritumoral cysts (*arrowheads*), which do not exhibit enhancement

Fig. 2.61 Spinal hemangioblastoma. (**a**) Sagittal postcontrast T1WI through the cervical and upper thoracic spine shows a brightly enhancing nodule (*arrow*) along the posterior surface of the spinal cord. There are adjacent intramedullary areas of low attenuation (*arrowheads*) corresponding to cystic change and edema. (**b**) Postcontrast axial T1WI through the mass (*arrow*) again demonstrates its peripheral location and bright enhancement

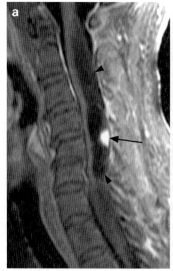

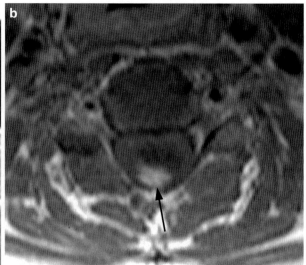

References

1. Osborn AG, et al. editors. Diagnostic imaging: brain. 2nd ed. Amirysis; 2009.
2. Osborn AG, et al. editors. Expert DDx brain and spine. 1st ed. Amirsys; 2010.
3. Bowen BC. 2nd ed. Spine imaging: case review. Mosby: Elsevier; 2007.
4. Cha S. Neuroimaging in neuro-oncology. Neurotherapeutics 2009;74:1319–22.
5. Rumboldt Z, Thurnher M, Gupta RK. Imaging of CNS infections. Semin Roentgenol 2007;42:62–91.

Case 3A
A 36-Year-Old Male with an Incidental Frontal Lesion

Cynthia T. Welsh

Clinical History

- 36-year-old male
- Pain in right eye
- CT of orbits demonstrated left frontal abnormality
- Normal neurologic exam

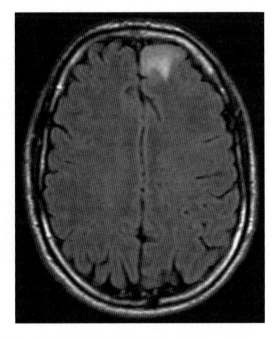

Fig. 3A.1 Axial MRI T2 FLAIR – left frontal lesion which appears to involve gray and white matters

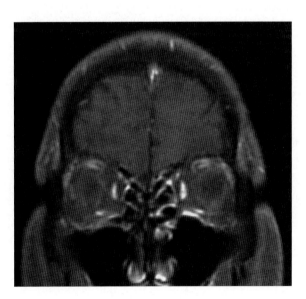

Fig. 3A.2 Coronal MRI T1 postcontrast – very little, if any, enhancement

C.T. Welsh (✉)
Department of Pathology and Laboratory Medicine,
Medical University of South Carolina, Charleston, SC 29425, USA
e-mail: welshct@musc.edu

C.T. Welsh (ed.), *Intra-Operative Neuropathology for the Non-Neuropathologist: A Case-Based Approach*,
DOI 10.1007/978-1-4419-1167-4_3, © Springer Science+Business Media, LLC 2012

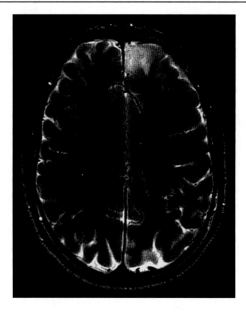

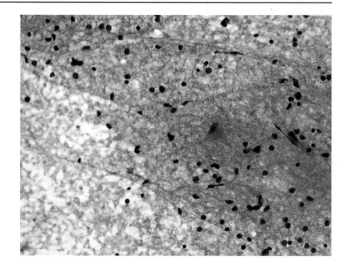

Fig. 3A.5 Smear (H&E high magnification) – gemistocyte

Fig. 3A.3 Axial MRI T2 – left frontal lesion which appears to involve gray and white matters

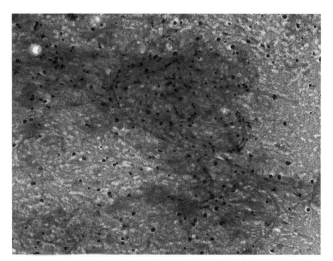

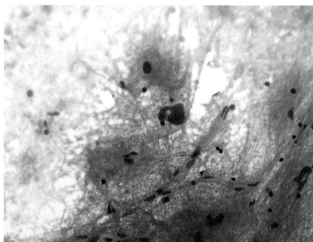

Fig. 3A.4 Smear (H&E low magnification) – tissue clumping

Fig. 3A.6 Smear (H&E high magnification) – "bare," irregular, hyperchromatic nucleus

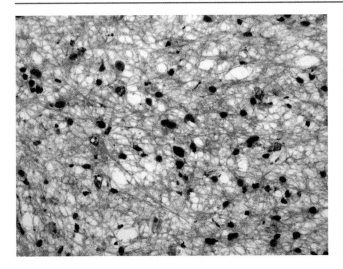

Fig. 3A.7 Frozen section (H&E high magnification) – "bare" irregular hyperchromatic nuclei

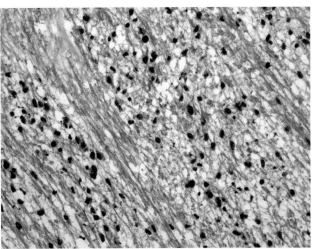

Fig. 3A.8 Frozen section (H&E high magnification) – increased cellularity with cell clusters infiltrating white matter tracts

What Is Your Diagnosis?

Figure Discussion

Scans

The coronal MRI pre- and postcontrast show no change (enhancement) in the left frontal tumor, just in vasculature next to the tumor, so only the postcontrast scan is shown. The tumor is much more apparent on the axial T2 scan, and the FLAIR sequence shows this is not just fluid, it is increased cellularity (Figs. 3A.1– 3A.3).

Pathology

Uneven smearing, mild increases in the number of cells with clustering of those cells, a change in the neurofibrillary background (looser than normal), and abnormal nuclei without visible individual cytoplasm/processes (bare nuclei) are all indications that not only is the tissue abnormal but also neoplastic. The processes are consistent with an astrocytic origin for the tumor cells. The cells are traveling along white tracts (Figs. 3A.4–3A.8).

Diagnosis: Low-Grade Astrocytoma

Low-grade tumors in adults tend to be associated with presenting seizure or long standing headache more often than high-grade tumors, or they may be an incidental finding as in this case. Tumors in adults tend to be supratentorial, and low-grade tumors are no exception. The most common low-grade tumors in adults, diffuse (fibrillary) astrocytomas (followed by the less common oligodendrogliomas), are infiltrative on MRI scans, bright on T_2 and FLAIR sequences, and do not enhance. This is in contrast to a number of the other low-grade gliomas (pleomorphic xanthoastrocytoma (PXA), ependymoma, pilocytic astrocytomas (PA), and ganglion cell tumors) which are distinct from surrounding neural tissue (Table 3A.1). Low-grade astrocytomas other than PA do not typically enhance or have necrosis. They often have cysts and are generally seen in younger patients. Glial tumors that infiltrate, such as fibrillary astrocytomas and oligodendrogliomas, may track along white matter tracts giving a thickened corpus callosum and/or internal capsule.

Intraoperatively, the age, clinical presentation, and fact that the tumor does not enhance should influence you heavily in favor of a low-grade process. White matter-based lesions tend to be astrocytic. The cortical based ones are often oligodendroglial, or dysembryoplastic neuroepithelial tumor (DNET). Or, particularly if grossly cystic, they may be PXA, ganglioglioma, or even pilocytic.

The low-grade astrocytoma will often be of low cellularity with the chief histologic differential being reactive gliosis or other low-grade tumor. The tissue will not smear as evenly as normal brain; clumping may be very similar to that of

Table 3A.1 Primary brain tumor configurations. Tumor growth patterns

Diffuse	Localized
Fibrillary astrocytoma	PXA
Oligodendroglioma	Pilocytic astrocytoma
Lymphoma	Ganglion cell tumor
	Ependymoma
	Choroid plexus tumor
	Subependymoma
	DNET
	Hemangioblastoma
	Neurocytoma
	SEGA

reactive brain. The neuroglial background will be abnormal. Neoplastic astrocytes have fewer, short, stubby processes than reactive astrocytes, or the processes are not apparent ("bare nuclei"). The cells tend to cluster, be less uniform, and/or be seen in numbers beyond the realms of just reactive (almost back to back). Nuclei are larger and more irregular than normal, or those seen in low-grade oligodendrogliomas. Some reactive lesions can actually show more nuclear atypia than low-grade neoplasms, but the cells also have lots of cytoplasm. Very little, or no, inflammation (especially neutrophils or macrophages) is usually seen. No high-grade features are present.

Differential Diagnosis: Gliosis

Gliosis (astrocytosis) is common to most processes in the brain. Reactive astrocytes make the brain appear too cellular and can easily be mistaken for tumor astrocytes. They make the tissue smear less evenly than normal brain, in a pattern very similar to low-grade tumor. The individual astrocytes may vary from a display of long, thin processes (Fig. 3A.9), which radiate evenly around the entire circumference of the nucleus to shorter, thicker, and fewer processes, which sometimes approach the changes seen in neoplasia. Early in the process, the cytoplasm becomes prominent next to the nucleus (gemistocytic change); later this perinuclear cytoplasm shrinks, but the cytoplasm in general remains more prominent than normal. The nuclear changes also show a large range, varying from small and oval to large, hyperchromatic, and irregular (once again simulating neoplasia). Nucleoli can become prominent in either reactive or neoplastic astrocytes. More reliable evidence (Table 3A.2) for the process being reactive includes the relatively even spacing of the cells (Fig. 3A.10), and the background (if present) of other cells such as macrophages, microglia, neutrophils, and (less useful) lymphocytes. Vessels are reactive (Fig. 3A.11) also as opposed to the complex vascular changes seen in tumors. Gliosis is

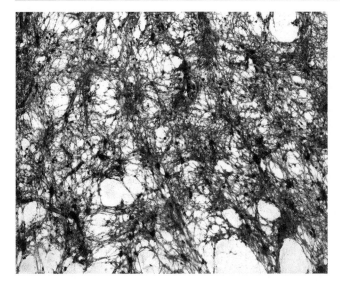

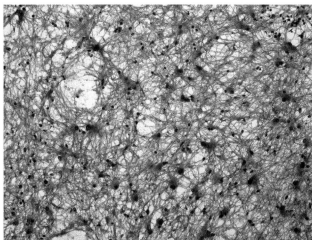

Fig. 3A.10 Histology – gliosis – even spacing of astrocytes

Fig. 3A.9 Smear – gliosis – long thin processes on astrocytes

Table 3A.2 Reactive brain versus neoplasm

	Gliosis	Diffuse astrocytoma
Radiologic findings		Loss of gray–white junction
Distribution of cells	Even	Irregular, clusters
Bare nuclei	No	Yes
Microcysts	Rare	Common
Macrophages	Depends on process	Rare
Other inflammatory cells	Depends on process	Rare
Satellitosis	No	Yes
Cell processes	Thin, long, uniform	Short, fat
More Rosenthal fibers than cells?	Frequent	Seldom
Calcification	No	Maybe
Vessels	Enlarged endothelial	Increased numbers cells

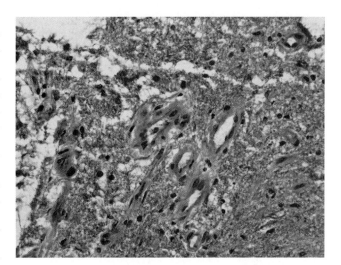

Fig. 3A.11 Histology – gliosis – reactive blood vessels

seen with infections, demyelinating processes (such as PML and MS), and vascular lesions (such as infarct). It is also seen adjacent to metastases and within/nearby oligodendrogliomas, so the fact that you see no tumor in the material at which you are presently looking, does not mean there is no tumor in the patient (a caveat to mention to the neurosurgeon).

Differential Diagnosis: Oligodendroglioma

Oligodendroglioma usually enters the differential when there are too many cells and they are not just reactive astrocytes or inflammatory cells. Around the edges of the tumor, where a few cells infiltrate the brain, is frequently the most difficult place to tell that the tumor is oligodendroglial. There are almost always reactive astrocytes present because of the brain infiltration. These also add to the cellularity, and may make the disease process appear to be astrocytic. Within the center of the low-grade oligodendroglioma there are evenly placed small cells (Table 3A.3) and small capillaries (Fig. 3A.12) around nests of cells ("chicken wire fencing") on tissue sections. The "haloes or fried eggs" so promptly diagnostic on permanent sections, are mostly an artifact of fixation, and usually won't be seen well on frozen sections. On smears the cells will have only a small rim of cytoplasm (Fig. 3A.13), if any, without the long processes of an

Table 3A.3 Cell distribution in brain

Process	Cell spacing
Normal/reactive astrocytes	Even
Diffuse astrocytoma	Clusters
Normal oligodendrocytes	Clusters, rows
Oligodendroglioma	Even spacing usually
	Occasionally cords

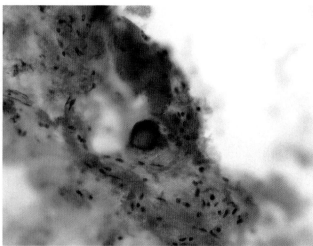

Fig. 3A.14 Smear – oligodendroglioma – microcalcification

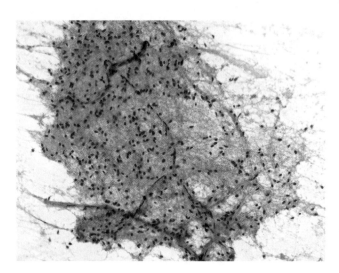

Fig. 3A.12 Smear – oligodendroglioma – fine capillaries small nuclei

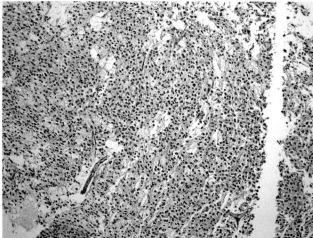

Fig. 3A.15 Histology – oligodendroglioma – microcysts

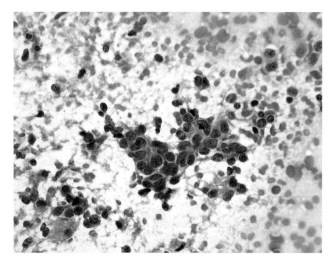

Fig. 3A.13 Smear – oligodendroglioma – sometimes a small rim of cytoplasm

many low-grade tumors, especially oligodendrogliomas. Satellitosis of tumor cells around neurons is more common than in astrocytic tumors. A few mitoses do not make an oligodendroglial tumor high grade, and hypercellular nodules are common in oligodendroglial tumors, so they shouldn't make you think high grade either.

Differential Diagnosis: Other Primary Low-Grade Glial Tumor

The appearance in these slides doesn't lend itself to as wide a differential as is actually possible with low-grade diffuse astrocytoma. If the morphology were gemistocytic, then you would want to know if the tumor were near the ventricle in a patient with Tuberous Sclerosis (high likelihood of a subependymal giant cell astrocytoma (SEGA)), or if the

astrocyte (often the cytoplasm is stripped off leaving bare nuclei). Nuclei having a large enough rim may be termed "mini- or microgemistocytes." The nuclei tend to be rounder, less irregular, and less pleomorphic than those of astrocytomas. Oligodendrogliomas commonly have calcifications (Fig. 3A.14), but these can be confused with corpora amylacea, bone dust, or other debris, and are not exclusive to oligodendrogliomas. Microcysts (Fig. 3A.15) are typical in

MRI showed a cyst with a peripheral nodule (possible PXA). SEGA (Fig. 3A.16) will have cells which appear somewhat neuronal admixed with the large astrocytic appearing cells. PXA have lipidized cells (Fig. 3A.17) and tend toward a degree of pleomorphism outside the usual bounds of gemistocytic astrocytomas. They are localized rather than infiltrative like all fibrillary tumors are (whether gemistocytic or not). Particularly, in certain locations where piloid astrocytes are common, the differential may include pilocytic astrocytoma. In a child with a posterior fossa astrocytic tumor, it will more often be pilocytic, but can be fibrillary (Fig. 3A.18) and yet appear spindled. The nuclei of pilocytic tumors are more spindled, and less irregular or hyperchromatic for the most part. The processes are hairlike ("piloid") or bipolar. Rosenthal fibers may be focal.

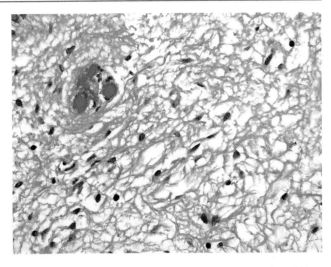

Fig. 3A.18 Histology – fibrillary astrocytoma – a suggestion of bipolar morphology

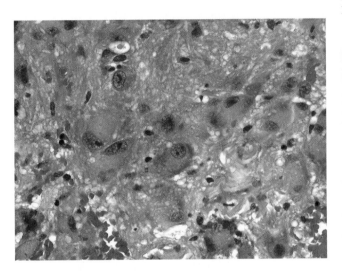

Fig. 3A.16 Histology – SEGA – large cells with variable cytoplasm; some eosniophilic, others with Nissl substance

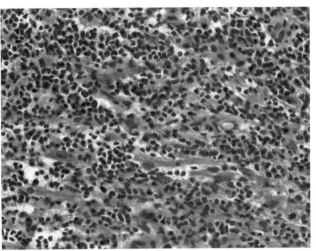

Fig. 3A.19 Histology – PCNSBL – infiltrating, monotonous, fairly small nuclei

Eosinophilic granular bodies are usually frequent. If large neurons are present, the question arises whether the neurons are part of normal gray matter infiltrated by tumor, or if the neurons are also neoplastic (ganglioglioma). Neoplastic neurons lack the organization of normal cortex rows and columns, they are often too large and/or too many for the location, and may be binucleate.

Differential Diagnosis: PCNSL

When cellularity is higher than seen in this case, or the nuclei are less angular, a primary lymphoma (Fig. 3A.19) may enter the differential diagnosis, particularly in an immunocompromised patient or someone elderly. A tumor location closer to ventricle than central white matter favors lymphoma.

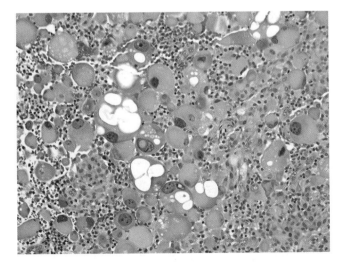

Fig. 3A.17 Histology – PXA – large cells with bizarre morphology and vacuoles

Perivascular cuffs of cells are seen best near the edges of the tumor. Primary CNS lymphomas are almost always large B-cell lymphomas (PCNSBL) with large vesicular nuclei, and usually fairly prominent nucleoli (which you will recognize as having a similar lymphoid character to the systemic large B-cell lymphomas with which you are familiar). Single cell death, which is uncommon in most glial tumors, is prominent in lymphomas. When the specimen is from the center of the tumor, the differential diagnosis is much more likely to be between lymphoma and some other high-grade tumor.

Bibliography

Low-Grade Astrocytoma

1 Lacoste-Collin L, d'Aure D, Aziza J, Quintyn ML, Uro-Coste E, Courtade-Saïdi M. Cerebrospinal fluid cytologic findings of a pleomorphic xanthoastrocytoma: a case report. Acta Cytol. 2010;54 Suppl 5:871–4.
2 Inagawa H, Ishizawa K, Hirose T. Qualitative and quantitative analysis of cytologic assessment of astrocytoma, oligodendroglioma and oligoastrocytoma. Acta Cytol. 2007;51(6):900–6.
3 Shukla K, Parikh B, Shukla J, Trivedi P, Shah B. Accuracy of cytologic diagnosis of central nervous system tumours in crush preparation. Indian J Pathol Microbiol. 2006;49(4):483–6.
4 Scarabino T, Giannatempo GM, Nemore F, Popolizio T, Stranieri A. Supratentorial low-grade gliomas. Neuroradiology. J Neurosurg Sci. 2005;49(3):73–6.2.
5 Shimizu H, Mori O, Ohaki Y, Kamoi S, Kobayashi S, Okada S, Maeda S, Naito Z. Cytological interface of diffusely infiltrating astrocytoma and its marginal tissue. Brain Tumor Pathol. 2005;22(2):59–74.
6 Browne TJ, Goumnerova LC, De Girolami U, Cibas ES. Cytologic features of pilocytic astrocytoma in cerebrospinal fluid specimens. Acta Cytol. 2004;48(1):3–8.
7 Han JH, Kim JH, Yim H. Intravascular lymphomatosis of the brain. Report of a case using an intraoperative cytologic preparation. Acta Cytol. 2004;48(3):411–4.
8 Yip M, Fisch C, Lamarche JB. AFIP archives: gliomatosis cerebri affecting the entire neuraxis. Radiographics 2003;23(1):247–53.
9 Cummings TJ, Hulette CM, Longee DC, Bottom KS, McLendon RE, Chu CT. Gliomatosis cerebri: cytologic and autopsy findings in a case involving the entire neuraxis. Clin Neuropathol. 1999;18(4):190–7.

Case 3B
A 40-Year-Old Female with New Onset Seizures

Cynthia T. Welsh

Clinical History

- 40-year-old female
- New onset seizures
- Right arm numbness
- History of pituitary adenoma (on medical treatment)
- Exam:
  - Decreased sensation right arm

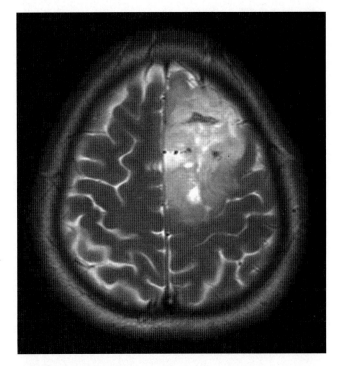

Fig. 3B.2 Axial MRI T2 – cortical involvement apparent

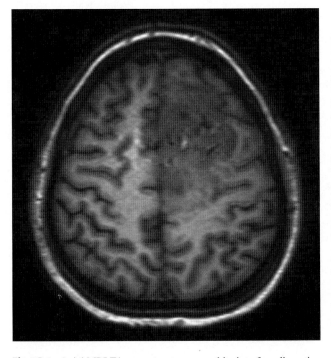

Fig. 3B.1 Axial MRI T1 precontrast – gray–white interface disruption in the left frontal lobe

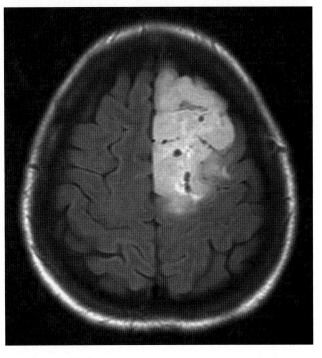

Fig. 3B.3 Axial MRI T2 FLAIR – cortical involvement apparent

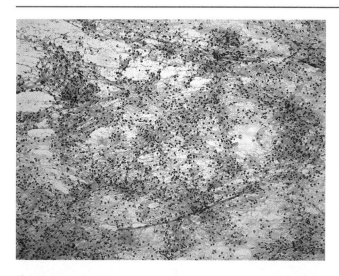

Fig. 3B.4 Smear (H&E low magnification) – microcysts, small nuclei, capillaries

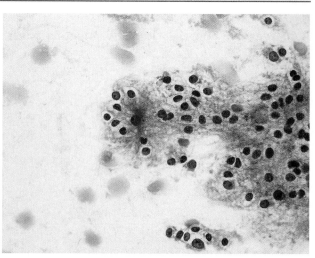

Fig. 3B.6 Touch preparation (H&E high magnification) – astrocyte surrounded by cells with cytoplasmic clearing

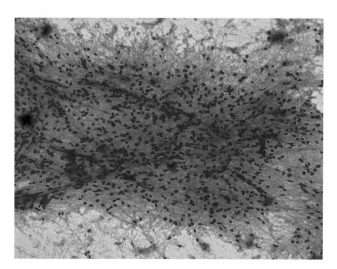

Fig. 3B.5 Smear (H&E low magnification) – small nuclei, background astrocytes, capillaries

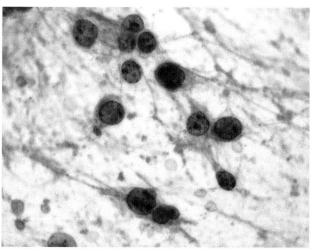

Fig. 3B.7 Smear (H&E high magnification) – small round nuclei, fine chromatin, and chromocenters

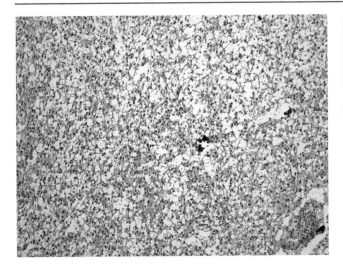

Fig. 3B.8 Frozen (H&E low magnification) – small nuclei, evenly spaced, perinuclear clearing

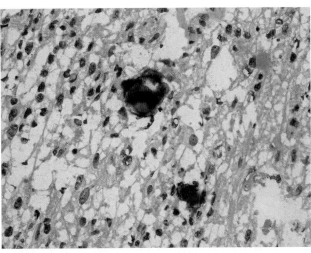

Fig. 3B.9 Frozen (H&E high magnification) – small nuclei, evenly scattered, microcalcifications, reactive astrocyte

What Is Your Diagnosis?

Figure Discussion

Scans

The tumor is dark on T1, and does not enhance (scan not included). It is more apparent on T2, and the cortical involvement is demonstrated particularly well on the FLAIR sequence (Figs. 3B.1–3B.3).

Pathology

Microcysts can break apart on smears done with too much pressure, but some of these are intact. The vascular pattern is predominantly that of increased capillary size vessels. Cytoplasmic clearing is seen on the touch preparation and a thin rim of cytoplasm on one smear. Calcifications are present. Nuclei are small and mostly round and seem evenly spaced on the low power histology. These are all findings consistent with an oligodendroglial origin for the tumor (Figs. 3B.4–3B.9).

Diagnosis: Oligodendroglioma

The low-grade oligodendroglioma centrally has evenly spaced small cells and small capillaries around nests of cells ("chicken wire fencing") on tissue sections. The "haloes or fried eggs" that we all equate with oligodendrogliomas, are mostly an artifact of fixation, and usually won't be well seen on frozen sections. On smears the cells will have only a small rim of cytoplasm, if any, without the long processes of an astrocyte (often the cytoplasm is stripped off leaving bare nuclei). The histologic differential diagnosis includes many other small cell processes, but the clinical history and radiologic findings sharply limit the *real* differential diagnosis. Patients with low-grade oligodendrogliomas are often young (although not always) and present with seizures. The cortical spread of the tumor that presumably accounts for the seizures can be seen on scans and should be a clue as to differential. Nuclei having a large enough rim may be termed "mini- or microgemistocytes." Oligodendroglial nuclei tend to be rounder, less irregular, and less pleomorphic than those of astrocytomas. Oligodendrogliomas commonly have microcalcifications (and larger calcifications may be seen on scans), but these can be confused with corpora amylacea, bone dust, or other debris, and can also be seen in other tumors (Table 3B.1). Microcysts are typical in many low-grade tumors, especially but not exclusively, oligodendroglial tumors (Table 3B.2). Satellitosis of tumor cells around neurons is so frequent, that the tumors often seem on scans to be cortically based, although once again oligodendrogliomas are not the only tumors to invade cortex (fibrillary astrocytomas do less commonly). Oligodendrogliomas commonly have nodules which are rather abruptly more cellular; these do not denote a tendency to higher grade. If no high-grade features are seen, the intraoperative diagnosis is most often "low-grade glioma." In sufficient numbers, mitoses would prompt you to say "high-grade glioma" intraoperatively in an astrocytoma, and complex microvascular changes may also. This is not true of oligodendrogliomas. So the nuclear details on smears (and sections), the vessels (are they all capillaries?), and the spacing of the cells (Table 3B.3) need to be considered carefully before upgrading the tumor.

Table 3B.1 Microcalcifications

Normal	
	Meninges
	Pineal
	Choroid plexus
Non-neoplastic conditions	
	Especially injury
	Particularly in children
Tumors	
	Oligodendroglioma – common in cortex
	Neurocytoma – common
	SEGA – common
	Astroblastoma
	Astrocytoma – occasional
	Ganglion cell tumors
	Ependymoma (particularly clear cell subtype)
	Pilocytic – occasional

Table 3B.2 Microcystic (all tumors!)

Meningioma
Pilocytic astrocytoma
Pilomyxoid astrocytoma
Oligodendroglioma
DNET
Ganglion cell tumors
Craniopharyngioma
PNST
Ependymoma
Subependymoma
Teratoma
Astroblastoma
Fibrillary astrocytoma – rarely

Table 3B.3 Cell distribution in brain

Process	Cell Spacing
Normal/reactive astrocytes	Even
Diffuse astrocytoma	Clusters
Normal oligodendrocytes	Clusters, rows
Oligodendroglioma	Even spacing usually
	Occasionally cords/ribbons

Differential Diagnosis: Gliosis (Astrocytosis)

Gliosis often enters the differential diagnosis for oligodendrogliomas because of the reactive astrocytes incited by the tumor cells infiltrating through brain. It is also seen with infections, demyelinating processes (such as PML and MS), and vascular lesions (such as infarct). The vacuolated cytoplasm of macrophages seen in many of these lesions can be mistaken for oligodendrocytes. Gliosis makes the tissue smear less evenly than normal brain, and more like low-grade tumor. It will make the tissue appear hypercellular. The individual astrocytes may vary from a display of long, thin processes, which radiate evenly around the entire circumference of the nucleus (Fig. 3B.10) to shorter, thicker, and fewer processes, which sometimes approach the changes seen in neoplasia. Early in the process, the cytoplasm becomes prominent next to the nucleus (gemistocytic change); later this perinuclear cytoplasm shrinks, but the cytoplasm in general remains more prominent than normal. The nuclear changes also show a large range, varying from small and oval to large, hyperchromatic, and irregular (once again simulating neoplasia). Nucleoli can become prominent in either reactive or neoplastic astrocytes. The nuclei are more angular than those of the low-grade oligodendroglioma. Evidence for the process being reactive includes the relatively even spacing of the astrocytes (Fig. 3B.11), and the background (if present) of other cells such as macrophages, microglia, neutrophils, and (less useful) lymphocytes. Vessels will be reactive in non-neoplastic gliosis (Fig. 3B.12) rather than show complex microvascular changes or the increased capillary architecture of an oligodendroglioma. The reactive astrocytes in an

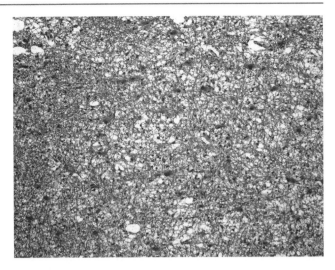

Fig. 3B.11 Histology – gliosis – even spacing of astrocytes and processes accentuated by ice crystal artifact

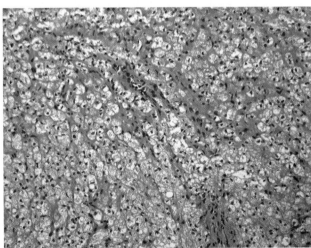

Fig. 3B.12 Histology – gliosis – reactive blood vessels in a sea of macrophages

oligodendroglioma should not lead you to call the tumor an oligoastrocytoma.

Differential Diagnosis: Normal White Matter

Normal oligodendrocytes appear in gray matter, are very numerous in white matter, and have a tendency toward clusters (Fig. 3B.13) and rows of cells that should not be confused with oligodendroglioma. We talk about using astrocyte spacing when we are comparing reactive with neoplastic; this does not apply to oligodendrocytes which normally form rows and groups. The first specimen from the neurosurgeon is actually often normal/reactive tissue on the way to the tumor.

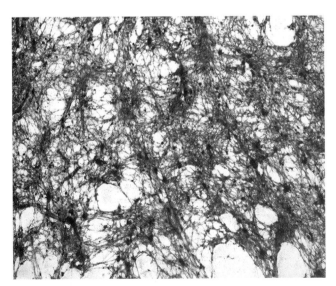

Fig. 3B.10 Smear – gliosis – long thin processes on clumps of astrocytes

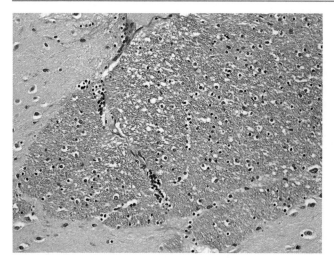

Fig. 3B.13 Histology – normal white matter – clusters of oligodendrocytes

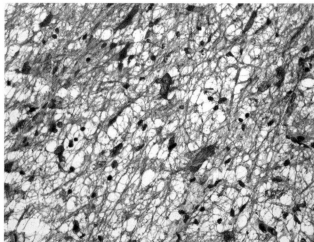

Fig. 3B.15 Histology – low-grade diffuse astrocytoma – large dark irregular "bare" nuclei

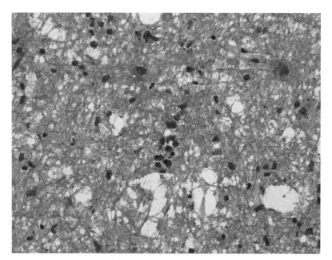

Fig. 3B.14 Histology – low-grade diffuse astrocytoma – clusters of cells

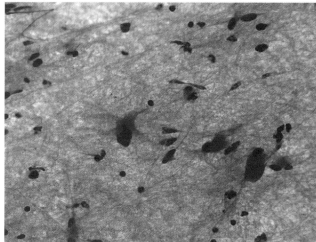

Fig. 3B.16 Smear – low-grade diffuse astrocytoma – few, short, broad processes

Differential Diagnosis: Low-Grade Diffuse Astrocytoma

Low-grade astrocytoma will often be of low cellularity and can be similar in appearance to the infiltrative edges of oligodendrogliomas. Unlike reactive astrocytes which remain fairly evenly spaced, or oligodendrogliomas which from low power also give you the impression of even spacing, neoplastic astrocytes tend to cluster (Fig. 3B.14). The nuclei are larger, and more hyperchromatic and irregular (Fig. 3B.15) than low-grade oligodendroglial nuclei. Astrocytic cells have processes which may show up well on frozen sections due to ice crystal artifact, but will definitely be very obvious on cytologic preparations (Fig. 3B.16). Astrocytomas have microcysts, microcalcifications, and secondary structures like satellitosis less often than oligodendrogliomas, but they

do still happen. Oligodendrogliomas are infiltrative tumors which incite an astrocytic reaction (gliosis). Do not confuse these astrocytes with neoplastic astrocytes and call the tumor an oligoastrocytoma. When no high-grade features are present, the intraoperative diagnosis is often "low-grade glioma" which is specific enough at that point.

Differential Diagnosis: Extraventricular Neurocytoma

Many neurocytomas are intraventricular, which should make you think of them in the differential (if you know the tumor location), but particularly when extraventricular, the differential diagnosis includes oligodendrogliomas. Neurocytomas can have haloes, microcalcifications, and small fairly round nuclei (Fig. 3B.17) like oligodendrogliomas. In comparison to oligodendroglioma, there is extra neuropil in neurocytomas and the tendency to make neuronal rosettes. The nuclei tend to be more uniformly round. Smears show the rosettes and clumps of neuropil, and you don't have the rim of cytoplasm that careful preparations from oligodendrogliomas can demonstrate. Because this tumor is localized rather than infiltrative, it doesn't have astrocytes within it, and is possible to totally remove, unlike oligodendrogliomas.

Differential Diagnosis: DNET

Dysembryoplastic neuroepithelial tumors (DNETs) have oligodendroglial appearing cells and microcysts (Fig. 3B.18). The neurons seen are not just trapped cortical neurons like in

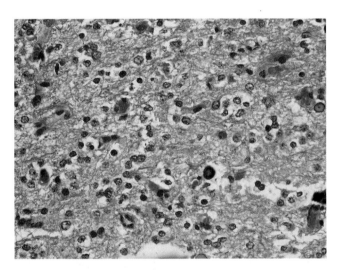

Fig. 3B.17 Histology – neurocytoma – cleared cytoplasm and microcalcifications

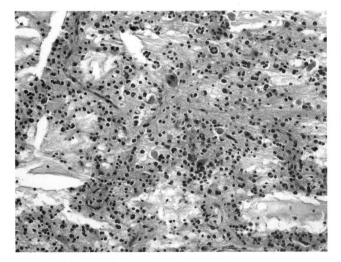

Fig. 3B.18 Histology – DNET – oligodendroglial-like cells, ganglion cells, and microcysts

oligodendrogliomas. DNET is potentially totally removable with no recurrence, so it can be important to differentiate from oligodendroglioma (which is neither of the above) during surgery. The patients are generally young and present with seizures also. The scans may show a pattern which you may also see on microscopy, of multiple nodules of microcystic change. The brain between the nodules will generally be less cellular than in other tumors.

Differential Diagnosis: PCNSL

Primary CNS lymphoma (PCNSL) usually has a periventricular location as opposed to oligodendroglioma which is cortical/subcortical, so knowing the location on scans helps you start differentiating between the two of them. There are sheets of back-to-back cells in the middle of both oligodendrogliomas and in PCNSL (Fig. 3B.19). Neither tumor cell usually has much cytoplasm in evidence. The cells are generally much larger in lymphomas (although they can appear deceivingly small in frozen sections), and nucleoli are usually prominent unlike oligodendroglioma. Low-grade oligodendroglioma does not have the necrosis that is typical for lymphoma. Lymphoma is not a surgical neoplasm, so intraoperative diagnosis allows for a shorter, less extensive procedure.

Differential Diagnosis: Pilocytic

Particularly in the cerebellum, pilocytic astrocytomas have cells within them that are oligodendroglial-like (Fig. 3B.20). In a child, in the posterior fossa, a pilocytic tumor would be much more common that an oligodendroglioma. Determination intraoperatively of the pilocytic nature of the tumor reassures the surgeon that gross total excision is a reasonable goal. Looking

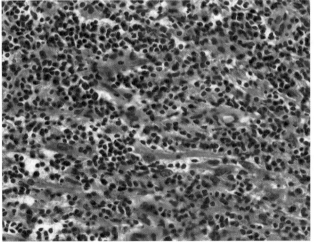

Fig. 3B.19 Histology – PCNSBL – infiltrating, monotonous, fairly small appearing cells

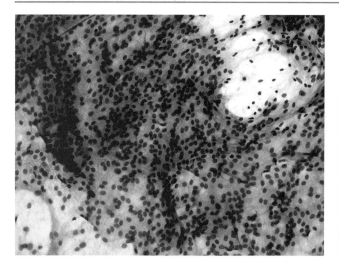

Fig. 3B.20 Smear – pilocytic – small round monotonous oligodendroglial-like nuclei

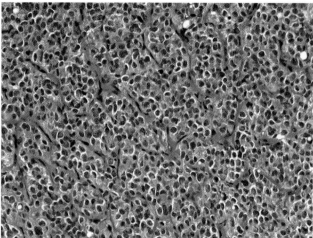

Fig. 3B.21 Histology – ependymoma – small nuclei with a suggestion of cytoplasmic clearing and increased capillaries

for the biphasic nature, hair-like "piloid" cells, and Rosenthal fibers helps to make the diagnosis and reassures the neurosurgeon that as complete an excision as possible is the correct course of action.

Differential Diagnosis: Ependymoma (Especially Clear Cell)

Clear cell ependymomas (Fig. 3B.21) have clear cells very similar to oligodendrogliomas and have microcalcifications like oligodendrogliomas. They tend more than other ependymomas to occur outside the ventricular system, but should appear more well circumscribed than oligodendrogliomas on scans. On either smears or frozen sections perivascular pseudorosettes (Fig. 3B.22) will be seen, but may be focal requiring extensive sampling. The nuclei of ependymal cells are generally more oval than oligodendrocytes, and the cytoplasm greater in volume and more eccentric (possibly actual processes). If the ependymal nature can be determined intraoperatively, the surgeon will be more likely to try to completely excise the tumor.

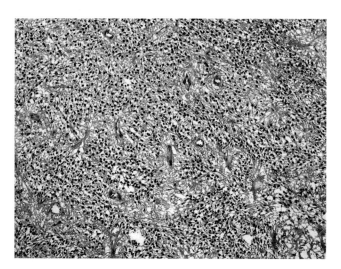

Fig. 3B.22 Histology – ependymoma – clearing around the small nuclei, but perivascular pseudorosettes

Differential Diagnosis: Small Cell Anaplastic

The small cell variant of fibrillary astrocytoma (Fig. 3B.23) has small cells with minimal cytoplasm and perinuclear haloes. The nuclei are often more oval than the typical elongate, irregular nuclei of astrocytomas. There is a brisker mitotic rate than in low-grade oligodendroglioma. The issue here will be more for eventual determination of the correct category for the tumor and subsequent type of appropriate molecular studies.

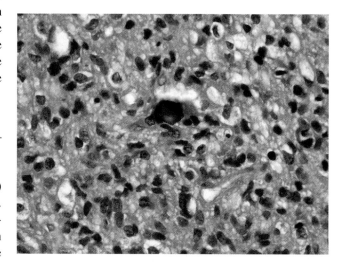

Fig. 3B.23 Histology – small cell anaplastic astrocytoma – irregular nuclei, cleared cytoplasm, microcalcification

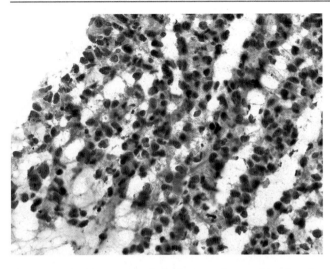

Fig. 3B.24 Histology – small cell glioblastoma – frozen artifact distorting the tissue, irregular pleomorphic nuclei, many mitoses

Differential Diagnosis: Glioblastoma

Pure oligodendroglioma with mitoses, complex microvascular changes, and necrosis is a WHO grade III tumor. A mixture of astrocytes with the oligodendrocytes makes the tumor glioblastoma with an oligodendroglial component, WHO grade IV, because the astrocytes are worse actors. The small cell variant of GBM (Fig. 3B.24) most closely resembles high-grade oligodendroglioma because the cells are smaller and packed closely together than typical for glioblastoma. Necrosis is often very focal. The diagnosis intraoperatively will be "high-grade glioma" and the final correct definition left for permanent sections.

Cautions

- Haloes are not always seen in oligodendrogliomas (so you will miss the diagnosis if you insist on seeing this feature).
- Oligodendrogliomas are not the only tumor with haloes (and don't forget normal cells can have haloes).
- Oligodendrogliomas are not automatically high grade based on mitoses and/or complex microvascular changes.

Bibliography

Oligodendroglioma

1 Kojima H, Mori K, Fukudome N, Iseki M, Shimizu S. Cytologic characteristics of intracytoplasmic refractile eosinophilic granular bodies in anaplastic oligodendroglioma: a case report. Acta Cytol. 2008;52(4):467–70.
2 Inagawa H, Ishizawa K, Hirose T. Qualitative and quantitative analysis of cytologic assessment of astrocytoma, oligodendroglioma and oligoastrocytoma. Acta Cytol. 2007;51(6):900–6.
3 Mitsuhashi T, Shimizu Y, Ban S, Ogawa F, Matsutani M, Shimizu M, Hirose T. Anaplastic oligodendroglioma: a case report with characteristic cytologic features, including minigemistocytes. Acta Cytol. 2007;51(4):657–60.
4 Koeller KK, Rushing EJ. From the archives of the AFIP: Oligodendroglioma and its variants: radiologic–pathologic correlation. Radiographics 2005;25:1669–88.
5 Park JY, Suh YL, Han J. Dysembryoplastic neuroepithelial tumor. Features distinguishing it from oligodendroglioma on cytologic squash preparations. Acta Cytol. 2003;47(4):624–9.
6 Monabati A, Kumar PV, Roozbehi H, Torabinezhad S. Cytologic findings in metastatic oligodendroglioma. Acta Cytol. 2003;47(4):702–4.
7 Park JY, Suh YL, Han J. Dysembryoplastic neuroepithelial tumor. Features distinguishing it from oligodendroglioma on cytologic squash preparations. Acta Cytol. 2003;47(4):624–9.
8 Anand M, Kumar R, Jain P, Gupta R, Ghosal N, Sharma A, Agarwal A, Sharma MC. Metastatic anaplastic oligodendroglioma simulating acute leukemia. A case report. Acta Cytol. 2003;47(3):467–9.
9 Goh SG, Chuah KL. Role of intraoperative smear cytology in the diagnosis of anaplastic oligodendroglioma. A case report. Acta Cytol. 2003;47(2):293–8.

Case 3C
A 74-Year-Old Female with Seizure, and Hemiparesis

Cynthia T. Welsh

Clinical History

- 74-year-old female
- Seizure, altered mental status
- Headache, left hemiparesis
- History ovarian cancer
- Exam:
    - Left facial droop
    - Left upgoing toe
    - Left side decreased sensation

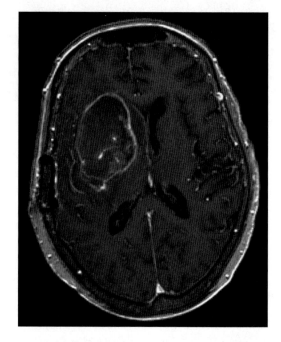

Fig. 3C.2 Axial MRI T1 postcontrast – ring enhancement

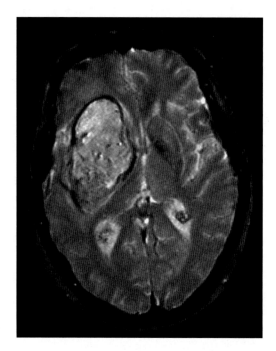

Fig. 3C.1 Axial MRI T2 – bright CSF and right hemisphere tumor

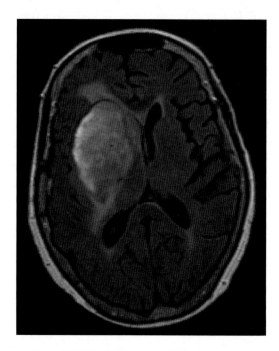

Fig. 3C.3 Axial MRI T2 FLAIR – dark CSF, but tumor remains bright

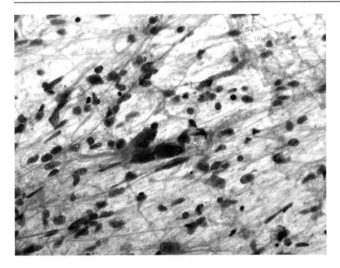

Fig. 3C.4 Smear (H&E high magnification) – large, hyperchromatic, irregular nuclei

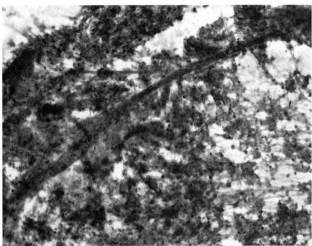

Fig. 3C.6 Smear (H&E high magnification) – necrosis

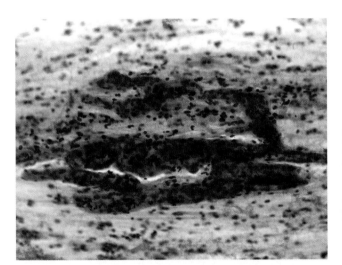

Fig. 3C.5 Smear (H&E high magnification) – complex microvascular change

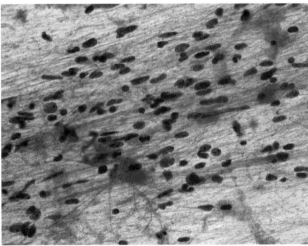

Fig. 3C.7 Smear (H&E high magnification) – mitosis

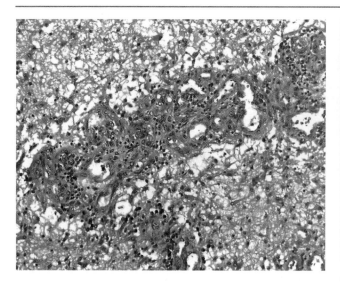

Fig. 3C.8 Frozen section (H&E low magnification) – complex micro-vascular change

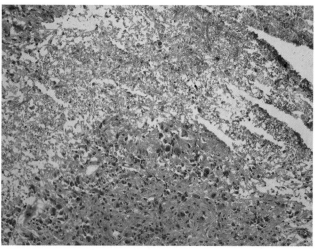

Fig. 3C.9 Frozen section (H&E low magnification) – necrosis

What Is Your Diagnosis?

Figure Discussion

Scans

The tumor enhances in approximately a ring with extra strands of contrast. The infiltration of tumor cells into brain outside of the main "mass" is illustrated by the bright signal on the FLAIR sequence (Figs. 3C.1–3C.3).

Pathology

The increased cellularity and numerous abnormal nuclei, most without individual cytoplasm (bare nuclei) are seen on both the smears and frozen section. The higher grade features of mitoses, complex microvasculature with increased vascular wall cellularity, and necrosis are also seen on both cytology and histology. The processes are consistent with an astrocytic neoplasm (Figs. 3C.4–3C.9).

Diagnosis: High-Grade Glioma

High-grade astrocytic tumors in adults can be seen at all ages, but tend to be more common with increasing age. The majority, as with most adult tumors, are supratentorial. On MRI scans, high-grade tumors enhance (Table 3C.1) and glioblastomas (GBM) usually enhance around necrosis (ring-enhancement). The differential diagnosis for the usual "ring-enhancing" lesion in an elderly adult consists of glioblastoma, metastasis, abscess, and lymphoma. During the intraoperative consultation, glial tumors are often designated as low or high-grade glioma (with grades 3 and 4 considered together) and astrocytic lumped with oligodendroglial as "glioma." Usually this information is enough for the neurosurgeon, although clinical research protocols may require more, such as being able to say "glioblastoma"; this may necessitate additional tissue. As glial tumors increase in grade, nuclear differences between astrocytic and oligodendroglial tumors start to blur. Vessels become more alike also. A higher grade is usually heralded microscopically by increased cellularity and mitoses first. Generally, the complex microvascular changes and necrosis are later than (in addition to) the mitoses. The mitoses, vascular changes, and necrosis can all be seen on both tissue sections and smears. If enough of the high-grade features (including necrosis) are present, and the tumor is definitely at least partly astrocytic then you can say it is a glioblastoma (we no longer use the term "multiforme").

Table 3C.1   Neoplastic enhancement on scans

Process	Patterns of enhancement
Glioblastoma	Irregular "shaggy" ring enhancement
Abscess	Thinner, more uniform ring enhancement
Lymphoma	Variable
Metastasis	Variable – much more edema than primary – more likely to hemorrhage

Pseudopalisading (Table 3C.2) around the necrosis is instantly recognizable but is not necessary for the diagnosis. There are many variants of glioblastoma such as giant cell, spindle cell, and small cell (which can be mixtures), and therefore many malignant metastatic tumors enter the histologic differential. They all have astrocytic differentiation, which may show better on smears, because the processes may be better defined. Even gemistocytic astrocytomas have processes. Astrocytic tumors have finer chromatin than metastases. They may have chromocenters, but nucleoli if present at all should be inconspicuous (as opposed to many metastases). Metastatic tumors form clumps and are often accompanied by at least some neuroglial tissue (which has a fine fibrillated background), and will give the impression of two populations of tissue if both are present on smears. The complex microvascular changes in a smear are spread out into arborizing structures rather than being all cropped at a single level as in a tissue section. In both preparations, tumor cells tend to cling to the vessels.

Therapeutic effects in previously diagnosed gliomas include macrophages becoming prominent, vessels becoming hyalinized and possibly less cellular appearing, necrosis in areas of tumor (or surrounding brain) which aren't very cellular (Fig. 3C.10), a paucity of mitoses, and occasionally increased numbers of truly bizarre astrocytic nuclei with intranuclear cytoplasmic pseudoinclusions.

Table 3C.2   Necrosis in brain lesions

Process	Differential features of necrosis
Glioblastoma Infarct	Dead vessels, pseudopalisading, coagulative Dead vessels
Metastasis	Pseudopapillary
Infection or infarct	Liquefactive, neutrophils and/or macrophages should raise non-neoplastic "flags"

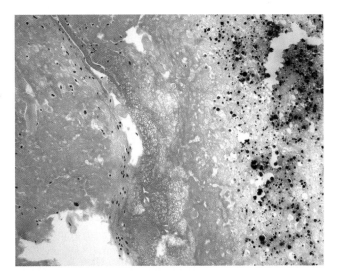

Fig. 3C.10 Histology – large areas of necrosis and a low level of cellularity after radiation therapy

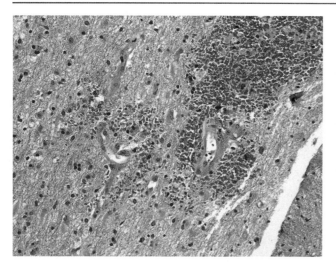

Fig. 3C.11 Histology – abscess – reactive vessels, inflammation

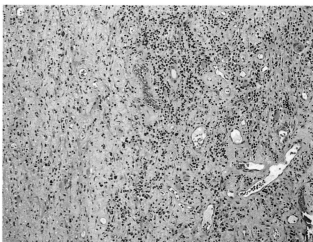

Fig. 3C.12 Histology – abscess – fibrotic wall

Differential diagnosis can also include acute multiple sclerosis (MS), particularly in younger females, which may show considerable necrosis. The lesions can be incredibly mitotically active in areas and show considerable reaction from surrounding vessels. But, this will be accompanied by macrophages, perivascular cuffs of lymphocytes and evenly scattered (though perhaps large and juicy) astrocytes.

Differential Diagnosis: Abscess

Abscesses also can have ring-enhancement, many mitoses, reactive blood vessels to be confused with tumor vessels, and bizarre astrocytes. But the vessels within the brain are pushed aside by an abscess and are reactive not "glomeruloid," the reactive astrocytes have abundant cytoplasm, the level of inflammation (Fig. 3C.11) is way over and above that of a glioblastoma, and the glioblastoma has a shaggier wall of enhancement. The fibrotic wall (Fig. 3C.12) of an abscess is not seen in gliomas. Significant numbers of neutrophils are almost never seen in primary glial tumors that have had no prior surgery, despite large areas of necrosis. Neutrophils and macrophages should make you think twice about calling the lesion a primary glioma.

Differential Diagnosis: High-Grade Oligodendroglioma

A few mitoses (Fig. 3C.13) and hypercellular nodules do not make an oligodendroglioma high grade. This can be one of the most problematic areas in frozen sections. You don't want to make a glioma with these features high grade unless you are sure it is astrocytic. All the high-grade features in a tumor which is purely oligodendroglial only make it WHO grade III. You also don't want to see dead or dying cells (Fig. 3C.14) and automatically assume it is a glioblastoma.

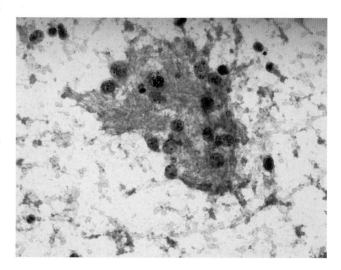

Fig. 3C.13 Smear – oligodendroglioma – mitoses

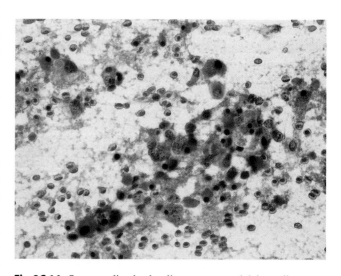

Fig. 3C.14 Smear – oligodendroglioma – scattered dying cells

Differential Diagnosis: Other Primary Lesions

PXA (pleomorphic xanthoastrocytoma) is a low-grade tumor with enough pleomorphism (Fig. 3C.15) that limited samples may be in the differential of glioblastoma. The PXA is non-infiltrative on radiology and tissue sections; if the boundary with adjacent brain isn't available in the frozen section, the MRI scans should clinch the issue. Necrosis is not present in low-grade PXA and mitoses are few despite the bizarre nature of the cells. Anaplastic PXA could remain in the differential however.

Primary CNS lymphomas may enhance, and if they do, it may be solid or ring-enhancement. They tend to be periventricular and can be multifocal. The peripheral zones of the tumor usually show "perivascular cuffing" which can be mistaken for "secondary structures of Scherer" – astrocyte tumor cells around vessels, or the other complex microvascular structures typical of high-grade glioma. The central areas with sheets of back-to-back cells show nuclei generally larger than those of glioblastoma (Fig. 3C.16) with less nuclear membrane irregularities and nucleoli that are conspicuous. Single cell necrosis is typical, something not classical for glioblastoma. Smears show the coarse chromatin, prominent nucleoli, and lack of processes better than frozen sections, and diff quik stains in particular highlight the lymphoid features.

PML (progressive multifocal leukoencephalopathy) can have some very bizarre astrocytes (Fig. 3C.17) and necrosis is expected. It is not unusual for PML to appear to follow white matter tracts like glial tumors do. But the macrophages and even distribution of the astrocytes should have you searching for infected oligodendroglial nuclei.

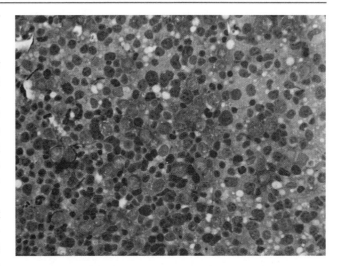

Fig. 3C.16 Histology – PCNSL – fairly round nuclei, many of them quite large, nucleoli

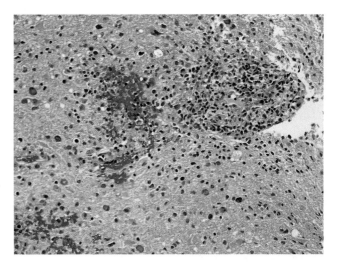

Fig. 3C.17 Histology – PML – large bizarre astrocytes, macrophages, perivascular lymphocytes

Differential Diagnosis: Metastasis

Metastases have a mass effect much more significant than their size alone would predict because of the surrounding edema, which is much more than seen with a primary tumor, in effect making their total volume higher than it would be otherwise. They have a pushing border, not the T_2-weighted infiltrative borders seen with primary tumors. Metastases tend to be multiple, but the smaller ones may not yet be in evidence at original presentation, while glioblastoma can have multiple sites of proliferation which mimic multifocality on scans. The T2 and FLAIR images distinguish metastases from glioblastoma. The metastasis will generally not show more than very little tendency to infiltrate at the edges on frozen sections and will show two cell populations (Fig. 3C.18) on smears; gliotic

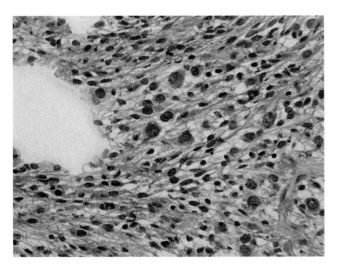

Fig. 3C.15 Histology – PXA – large pleomorphic astrocytes

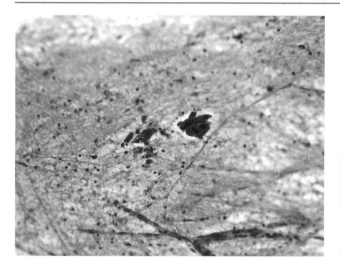

Fig. 3C.18 Smear – metastasis – two cell populations

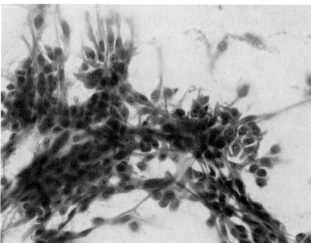

Fig. 3C.20 Smear – metastasis – nucleoli, coarse chromatin

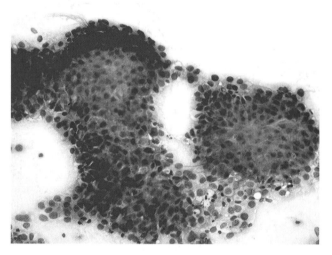

Fig. 3C.19 Smear – metastasis – balls of cells

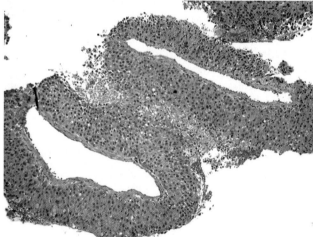

Fig. 3C.21 Histology – metastasis – "pseudopapillary" necrosis

brain, and balls of tumor usually (Fig. 3C.19). Metastases have coarser chromatin than astrocytic tumors. Many metastases have prominent nucleoli (Fig. 3C.20) as compared to astrocytic tumors which may have chromocenters, but nucleoli if present at all are usually inconspicuous. The pattern of necrosis for many metastases is a pseudopapillary one (Fig. 3C.21) as opposed to the pseudopalisading on high-grade glial lesions. The necrosis in metastases often incites an acute inflammatory reaction (Fig. 3C.22) and macrophage infiltration, unlike primary glial tumor necrosis, which usually does not cause much inflammatory response.

Differential Diagnosis: Infarct

Infarcts may be mistaken on CT for tumor. At some point in time they will enhance around the central necrosis. The macrophages present at this point in time, or red neurons

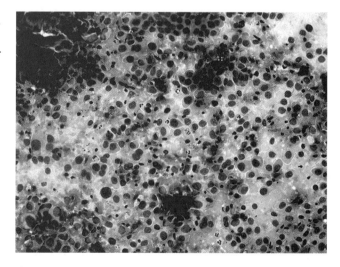

Fig. 3C.22 Smear – metastasis – inflammation and tumor cells

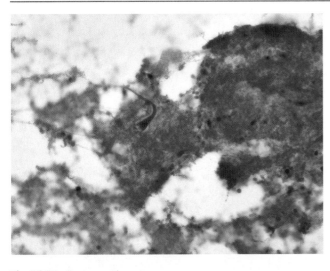

Fig. 3C.23 Smear – red neuron

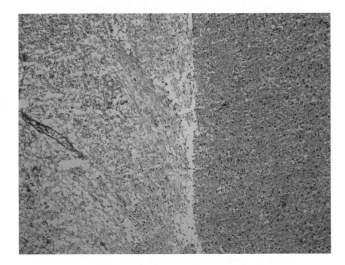

Fig. 3C.24 Histology – dead vessels

(Fig. 3C.23) if it is earlier (and they are present) will make this diagnosis for you. The vessels are reactive, not the complex microvascular changes seen around necrosis in high-grade glial tumors. Dead vessels will be seen within the necrosis (Fig. 3C.24).

Cautions

- GBM is glioblastoma (no longer multiforme).
- Macrophages in any significant numbers should always make you take a step back and reconsider whether you are looking at tumor.
- Neutrophils are also an unusual accompaniment to primary glial tumor.

Bibliography

High-Grade Glioma

1 Takei H, Florez L, Bhattacharjee MB. Cytologic features of subependymal giant cell astrocytoma: a review of 7 cases. Acta Cytol. 2008;52(4):445–50.
2 Amr SS, Al-Tawfiq JA. Aspiration cytology of brain abscess from a fatal case of cerebral phaeohyphomycosis due to Ramichloridium mackenziei. Diagn Cytopathol. 2007;35(11):695–9.
3 Kim SH, Lee KG, Kim TS. Cytologic characteristics of subependymal giant cell astrocytoma in squash smears: morphometric comparisons with gemistocytic astrocytoma and giant cell glioblastoma. Acta Cytol. 2007;51(3):375–9.
4 Chen KT. Crush cytology of pleomorphic xanthoastrocytoma. Acta Cytol. 2006;50(4):446–8.
5 Hernandez O, Zagzag D, Kelly P, Golfinos J, Levine PH. Cytological diagnosis of cystic brain tumors: a retrospective study of 88 cases. Diagn Cytopathol. 2004;31(4):221–8.
6 Goel S, Kapila K, Sarkar C, Verma K. Cytodiagnosis of anaplastic astrocytoma with metastasis to the cerebrospinal fluid in a neonate – a case report. Neurol India. 2003;51(2):276–7.
7 Collaço LM, Tani E, Lindblom I, Skoog L. Stereotactic biopsy and cytological diagnosis of solid and cystic intracranial lesions. Cytopathology 2003;14(3):131–5.
8 Masuda K, Yutani C, Akutagawa K, Yamamoto S, Hatsuyama H, Ishibashi-Ueda H, Imakita M, Manaka H, Takahashi J, Nagata I. Cerebral primitive neuroectodermal tumor in an adult male. A case report. Acta Cytol. 2000;44(6):1050–8.
9 Deshpande AH, Munshi MM. Rhinocerebral mucormycosis diagnosis by aspiration cytology. Diagn Cytopathol. 2000;23(2):97–100.
10 Kobayashi S, Hirakawa E, Haba R. Squash cytology of pleomorphic xanthoastrocytoma mimicking glioblastoma. A case report. Acta Cytol. 1999;43(4):652–8.

Case 3D
A 50-Year-Old Male with Seizure and Unilateral Weakness

M. Timothy Smith

Clinical History

- 50-year-old man
- Long history of tobacco use
- Decreased mentation, unilateral weakness, and new onset seizures
- Exam – right hemiparesis

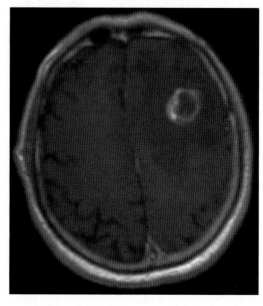

Fig. 3D.2 Axial MRI T1 postcontrast – small anterior left lesion brightly enhancing with a large amount of surrounding edema (which is darker than the brain parenchyma)

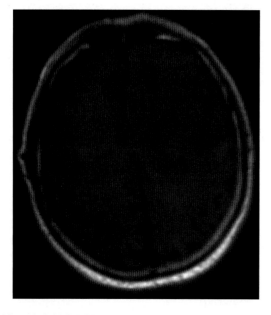

Fig. 3D.1 Axial MRI T1 precontrast – large left hemisphere anterior lesion

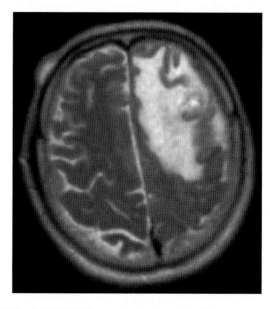

Fig. 3D.3 Axial MRI T2 – vasogenic edema in white matter

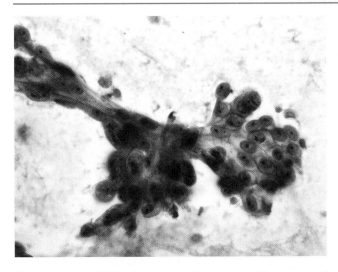

Fig. 3D.4 Smear (H&E stain high magnification) – papillary groups of cells with distinct cell borders and obvious nucleoli

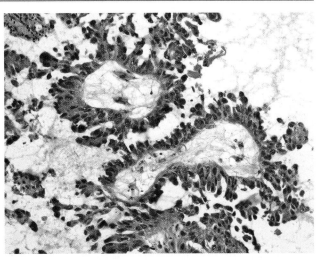

Fig. 3D.6 Frozen section (H&E high magnification) – papillary groups of cells with irregular appearing, hyperchromatic, pleomorphic nuclei, but no obvious mitoses

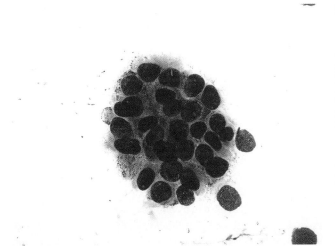

Fig. 3D.5 Smear (DQ stain high magnification) – ball of cells, fairly monotonous appearing nuclei with nucleoli

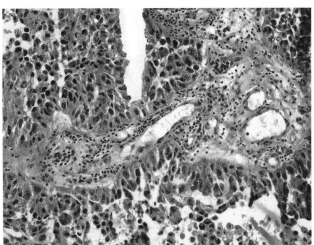

Fig. 3D.7 Frozen section (H&E high magnification) – high N/C ratio, pseudostratification of nuclei, with some nuclei at the surface of the cell (hobnail), rare mitoses

What Is Your Diagnosis?

Figure Discussion

Scans

The "mass effect" is a combination of the actual mass (small) and the prominent edematous reaction to the mass, which combine to cause symptoms when the tumor is still relatively small. The ring enhancement outlines an undoubtedly necrotic center (Figs. 3D.1–3D.3).

Pathology

Metastases have as many patterns as their original tumors do. This one is papillary with a high N/C ratio, prominent nucleoli, and well-defined (epithelial) cell borders which are all demonstrated nicely on cytologic preparations. The cells also form balls of cells on the smears as adenocarcinomas so often do (no matter where they are). There are no processes. The histology shows the fibrovascular cores, mitoses, and lymphocytic infiltrate. There is no fine fibrillar background suggesting brain in the tumor sections (Figs. 3D.4–3D.7).

Diagnosis: Metastatic Tumor

Cerebral metastases in adults are common and may be the first sign of a systemic primary. Common primary sources are lung, breast, gastrointestinal tract, kidney, prostate gland, skin (melanoma), and thyroid gland. Most metastasize to the brain proper, whereas prostatic carcinoma seldom goes to brain parenchyma, but instead goes to adjacent bone and affects brain/spinal cord after growth and compression. Metastases in the vertebral column are commonly breast carcinomas, prostate carcinomas, and lymphoma. Spinal cord parenchymal metastases are unusual. MRI appearances are variable, but multiple lesions are a significant clue. Proper subclassification of metastases can await permanent sections. Systemic malignancies may affect the subarachnoid space only, producing carcinomatous meningitis. These originate from lung, breast, and stomach. Metastases are often multifocal and well circumscribed. Pathologists are asked to intraoperatively distinguish between glial and nonglial malignancies or lymphoma. Frozen sections reveal the nonglial nature of the metastatic tumor, i.e., no fine fibrillar, vacuolated background. Deposits of metastatic carcinoma in the brain usually form groups of tumor cells that are clearly separate from the adjacent reactive neuropil. Carcinoma cells do not normally infiltrate in single cell fashion in the brain as do the cells of malignant gliomas. The notable exception is melanoma, a tumor that may infiltrate in single cell fashion, possibly because it is also of neuroectodermal origin. Papillary, glandular, or other patterns may be present recapitulating the pathology of the primary. Necrosis can be extensive (Table 3D.1).

Cytological features on smears are expectedly variable depending on the primary source and resemble the FNA appearance of the primary. Epithelial cells maintain some

Table 3D.1 Necrosis in brain lesions

Process	Differential features of necrosis
Glioblastoma	Dead vessels, pseudopalisading, coagulative
Infarct	Dead vessels
Metastasis	Pseudopapillary, sometimes single cell death prominent
Infection or infarct	Liquefactive, neutrophils, and/or macrophages should raise non-neoplastic "flags"

cohesiveness, and may make balls of cells but also disperse in small groups and single cells at the edges of the larger groups. Some tumors cling to the sides of tumor vessels, without the cytoplasmic processes of primary glial tumors. A background malignant necrotic diathesis is usually present and multiple kinds of inflammatory cells are a common response. Cytoplasm quantity is expectedly variable and cytoplasmic borders are more distinct than with glial cells. Glial-like processes seldom extend from tumor cells. Tumor nuclei are large, often with central nucleoli (unusual for glial cells), and chromatin is coarser than in glial cells. Mitoses are easily found. A fine glial fibrillary background is lacking within metastases. Separate clumps of reactive glial tissue may be present, giving the impression of two separate cell populations.

Specific features of some tumors may be found. For example, the nuclear molding of small cell carcinoma, or the clear cells and vascular pattern of renal cell carcinoma may be present. Melanin may be seen in the discohesive cells of metastatic melanoma. Gland formation or cytoplasmic keratin can often be identified in metastases. Small cell lung carcinoma metastases will morphologically mimic primitive neuroectodermal tumors (PNETs). A small cell PNET-like tumor in the cerebrum of an adult is most likely a metastasis but a small cell PNET-like tumor in the cerebellum of a child is usually a medulloblastoma. A small blue cell tumor in the hemispheres can be metastatic small cell carcinoma or a cerebral neuroblastoma. A deferred diagnosis intraoperatively is appropriate; immunohistochemistry and correlation with the clinical information will be critical to the final diagnosis. Rhabdomyosarcoma occurs rarely as a primary tumor in the brain as well as the meninges. Ewing's sarcoma and neuroblastoma may metastasize to the skull.

Differential Diagnosis: Lymphoma

Lymphomas of the brain can be either secondary or primary making about 1% of brain tumors. Primary CNS lymphomas were once rare, but now are much more common, being associated with the AIDS epidemic, transplant patients, chemotherapy patients, and other situations of immunocompromise (including age) so history is important. In order of frequency, the cerebrum, cerebellum, and epidural space are involved, often with multiple lesions. Of hematopoietic tumors, plasma cell dyscrasias predominate in skull and vertebrae. MRI often

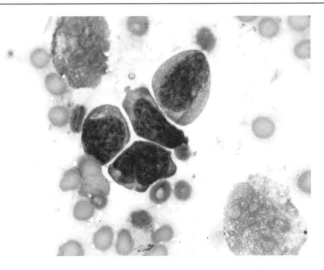

Fig. 3D.8 Touch preparation – PCNSBL – single large cells with large nuclei, smudged nuclei in the background

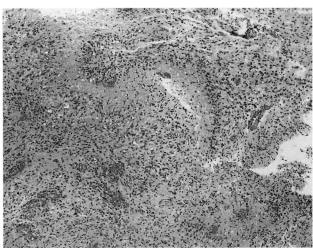

Fig. 3D.9 Histology – glioblastoma – pseudopalisading necrosis

shows periventricular involvement with primary lymphomas but subarachnoid involvement with systemic lymphomas. T1-weighted MRIs are usually hypointense. Lymphoma may be multifocal and enter the differential diagnosis of metastases. Squash cytology displays sheets of lymphoid cells transected by mildly hyperplastic vessels. The individual cells are those of the lymphoid series showing follicular center cell or cleaved morphology. Most are B cell lymphomas. Plasmacytoid features may be present. Lymphomas possess cytology distinct from metastases, small cell carcinoma, and glial tumors that is best appreciated on cytologic preparations. Touch preparations from lymphomas (Fig. 3D.8) will show single cells and may show smudged nuclei characteristic of lymphoma/leukemia. Frozen sections have the typical architectural pattern of perivascular lymphoid cuffing, especially toward the edges of the tumor. The lymphoid infiltrates permeate the vessel walls, forming tumor aggregates that may show necrosis. Recognizing intraoperatively that the tumor is a lymphoma allows for flow cytometry and appropriately stops the surgery at biopsy, rather than resection.

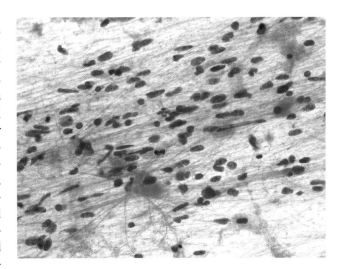

Fig. 3D.10 Smear – high-grade glioma – fine chromatin, mitoses, reactive astrocytes

tumor. Recognition of the glial background and infiltrative nature intraoperatively allows you to appropriately classify these tumors as primary malignancies.

Differential Diagnosis: High-Grade Glioma

High-grade glioma is infiltrative on scans and on tissue sections, in contrast to metastases. When the complex microvascular changes are glomeruloid, the diagnosis favors glioma. When there is "pseudopalisading" around the necrosis (Fig. 3D.9), rather than "pseudopapillary" structures formed by the necrosis, glioma is more likely. Astrocytic tumors have finer chromatin (Fig. 3D.10) than metastases. They may have chromocenters, but nucleoli if present at all should be inconspicuous (as opposed to many metastases). Glioblastomas can appear multifocal by imaging and can rarely have epithelial metaplasia. Their predominant morphology will display a glial fibrillary background identifying the nature of the

Differential Diagnosis: Malignant Dural Tumors

Malignant meningioma (Fig. 3D.11) can assume spindled, very epithelioid, or clear cell morphologies causing some difficulty in distinguishing it from a dural carcinoma metastasis. Secretory meningiomas can also resemble adenocarcinomas but usually lack the usual pleomorphism, necrosis, mitotic rate, and nucleoli of a metastasis. The herringbone pattern of fibrosarcoma is frequent in meningiomas as they become more malignant. An extra frozen section from a different area may reveal a more typical meningioma pattern or psammoma bodies, thus revealing the tumor's true nature.

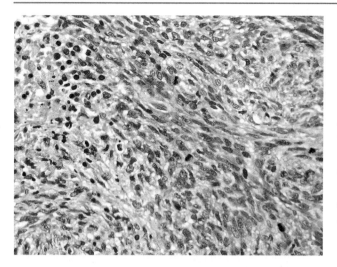

Fig. 3D.11 Histology – malignant meningioma – cellular pleomorphic tumor with necrosis and mitoses

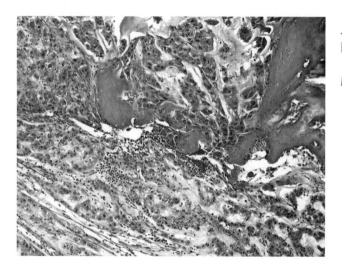

Fig. 3D.12 Histology – chordoma – two cell types (one eosinophilic, the other vacuolated) in a myxoid matrix within bone

Differential Diagnosis: Primary Bone Tumors Versus Base of Skull Mets

Chordomas are slowly growing extradural tumors of bone that arise from remnants of notochord at extreme ends of the neuraxis, usually the clivus or the sacrum. Rarely do they originate along the pharynx or thoracic vertebrae. Chondrosarcoma and chordoma occur in similar locations and have passing similarities on histology also. The cytology of chordoma smear preparations shows epithelioid cells singly, and in small groups, and rows and chains of cells floating in pools of basophilic mucoid material. Bubbly or vacuolated cytoplasm (physaliphorous) may be poorly represented in smears. Nuclei are bland and mitoses are rare. The tumor usually has a lobular pattern created by fibrous septae partitioning the extracellular mucoid material (Fig. 3D.12).

The extracellular mucoid material varies greatly in quantity, so some chordomas may be mostly solid. The vacuolated cytoplasm can resemble that of adenocarcinomas, but the pleomorphism, atypia, and malignant diathesis of adenocarcinoma are lacking.

Cautions

- History can sometimes help you recognize the tumor pattern you are seeing (despite the frozen artifacts).
- Multiple lesions on scans are most often metastatic.
- Melanomas can be somewhat infiltrative.

Bibliography

Metastatic Tumor

1 Barresi V, Tuccari G, Alafaci C, Caffo M. Importance of intraoperative cytology in the definition of cystic solitary brain lesions. Diagn Cytopathol. 2010;38(11):854–6.
2 Sioutopoulou DO, Kampas LI, Gerasimidou D, Valeri RM, Boukovinas I, Tsavdaridis D, Destouni CT. Diagnosis of metastatic tumors in cerebrospinal fluid samples using thin-layer cytology. Acta Cytol. 2008;52(3):304–8.
3 Han L, Bhan R, Johnson S, Zak I, Husain M, Al-Abbadi MA. Leptomeningeal metastasis in a patient with squamous cell carcinoma of the uterine cervix: Report of a case and review of the literature. Diagn Cytopathol. 2007;35(10):660–2.
4 Kobayashi TK, Bamba M, Ueda M, Nishino T, Muramatsu M, Moritani S, Katsumori T, Oka H, Hino A, Fujimoto M, Kushima R. Cytologic diagnosis of brain metastasis from hepatocellular carcinoma by squash preparation. Diagn Cytopathol. 2006;34(3): 227–31.
5 Hernandez O, Zagzag D, Kelly P, Golfinos J, Levine PH. Cytological diagnosis of cystic brain tumors: a retrospective study of 88 cases. Diagn Cytopathol. 2004;31(4):221–8.
6 Glosová L, Dundr P, Effler J, Růzicková M. Gallbladder carcinoma cells in cerebrospinal fluid as the first manifestation of a tumor. A case report. Acta Cytol. 2003;47(6):1087–90.
7 Parwani AV, Taylor DC, Burger PC, Erozan YS, Olivi A, Ali SZ. Keratinized squamous cells in fine needle aspiration of the brain. Cytopathologic correlates and differential diagnosis. Acta Cytol. 2003;47(3):325–31.
8 Deshpande AH, Munshi MM. Rhinocerebral mucormycosis diagnosis by aspiration cytology. Diagn Cytopathol. 2000;23(2): 97–100.
9 Monabati A, Kumar PV, Kamkarpour A. Intraoperative cytodiagnosis of metastatic brain tumors confused clinically with brain abscess. A report of three cases. Acta Cytol. 2000;44(3): 437–41.
10 Horn KD, Richert CA, Rajan PB, Bastacky SI, Peterson AB, Barnes EL. Cytologic findings of metastatic mucin-secreting adenocarcinoma of brain from parotid gland primary. Cytopathology 1999;10(5):341–4.

Case 3E
A 70-Year-Old Male with Dense Hemiparesis and History of Kidney Transplant

M. Timothy Smith

Clinical History

- 70-year-old man
- Progressive development of a dense hemiparesis over a period of 4 days

- Kidney transplant 3 years ago
- Exam – unoriented ×3, receptive aphasia

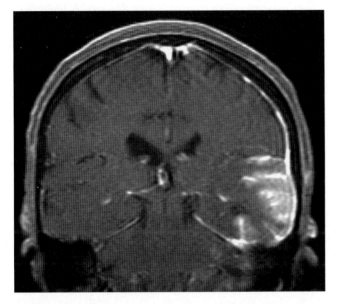

Fig. 3E.1   Coronal MRI T1 postcontrast – left temporal lobe enhancement in a "gyral" pattern

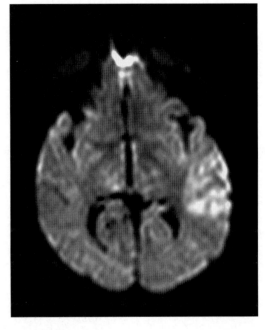

Fig. 3E.3   Axial MRI diffusion – demonstrating no fluid movement (bright) in these gyral areas

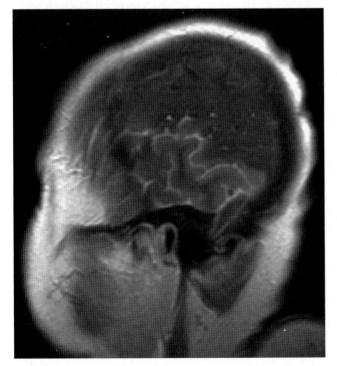

Fig. 3E.2   Sagittal MRI T1 postcontrast – enhancement in a "gyral" pattern

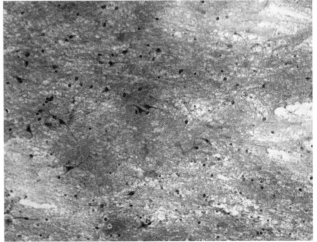

Fig. 3E.4   Smear (H&E low magnification) – minor clumping of tissue with scattered cells bearing red cytoplasm

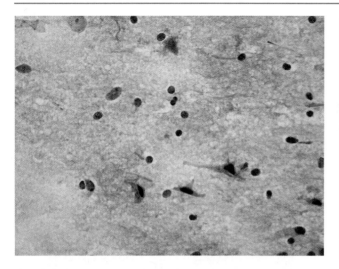

Fig. 3E.5 Smear (H&E high magnification) – a closer view of those same cells

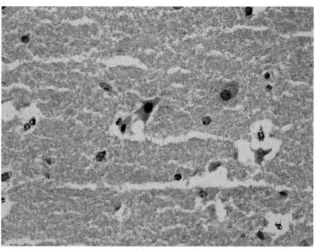

Fig. 3E.7 Frozen section (H&E high magnification) – a closer view of those same cells with the red cytoplasm

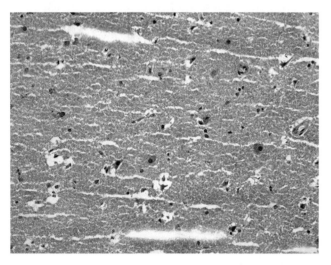

Fig. 3E.6 Frozen section (H&E low magnification) – those same cells scattered in the tissue section

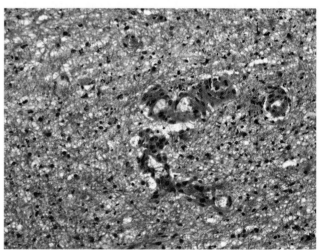

Fig. 3E.8 Frozen section (H&E low magnification) – prominent vessels with large endothelial cells

What Is Your Diagnosis?

Figure Discussion

Scans

The surgery was performed because the enhancement was felt to be leptomeningeal (suggesting possible tumor or infection) rather than gyral (indicating ischemia). The diffusion scan, however, supports the impression of ischemic change (Figs. 3E.1–3E.3).

Pathology

Obviously all cells in the CNS with red cytoplasm are not gemistocytic. These cells have a distinctly pyramidal morphology. The change seen in the vessels is reactive with endothelial hyperplasia (Figs. 3E.4–3E.8).

Diagnosis: Infarct

Occasionally, as in this instance, red neurons will be the diagnostic feature in an infarct. They can be mistaken for astrocytes. In contrast to the pyramidal shape of the eosinophilic neurons, gemistocytic astrocytes (Fig. 3E.9) are more globular, and multiple processes may be more or less apparent. More often, the patient is in the subacute stage of an infarct when someone clinically begins to suspect that it may be something other than "stroke." The pathology at this time usually enters into the "necrosis of various causes" set of differential diagnoses (Table 3E.1). One of the most useful cells to look for and lead to a non-neoplastic diagnosis in the case of subacute infarct will be the macrophage (Fig. 3E.10). On frozen sections, macrophage cell borders become indistinct, and their cytoplasm fairly clear like ice crystal artifact or oligoden-

Table 3E.1 Necrosis in brain lesions

Process	Differential features of necrosis
Glioblastoma	Dead vessels, pseudopalisading, coagulative
Infarct	Dead vessels
Metastasis	Pseudopapillary, sometimes single cell death prominent
Infection or infarct	Liquefactive, neutrophils, and/or macrophages should raise non-neoplastic "flags"

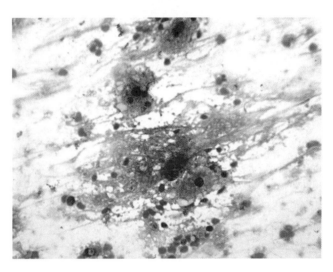

Fig. 3E.10 Smear – subacute infarct – macrophages and an astrocyte

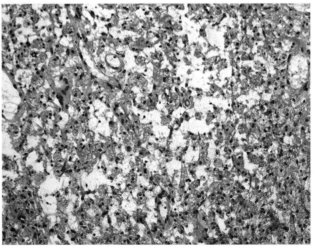

Fig. 3E.11 Histology – subacute infarct – macrophages stuffed with debris

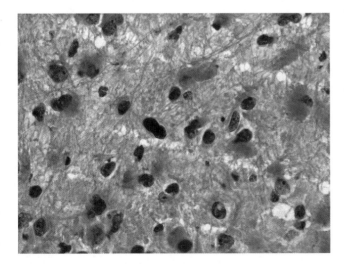

Fig. 3E.9 Histology – glioma – some of the astrocytes have obvious globular eosinophilic cytoplasm (gemistocytes)

droglial cells with nuclei small and round like oligodendroglial cells. These cells may be difficult to recognize on frozen sections unless they are stained well (Fig. 3E.11), making cytologic preparations invaluable. On cytology, macrophages show a low N/C ratio, foamy/granular cytoplasm, debris/

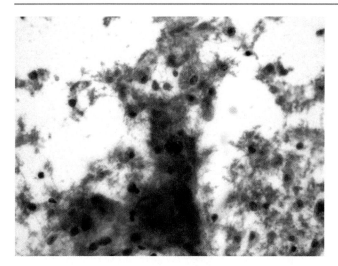

Fig. 3E.12 Smear – subacute infarct – macrophages with occasional hemosiderin

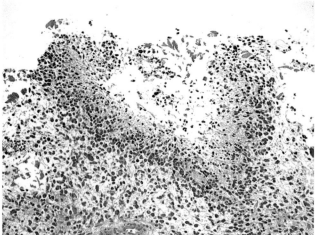

Fig. 3E.13 Histology – GBM – piling up of nuclei around the edges of an area of necrosis

hemosiderin in cytoplasm (Fig. 3E.12), and small round monomorphic nuclei with chromatin pattern less dense than oligodendroglial nuclei.

Differential Diagnosis: Glioblastoma

In an older adult, high-grade glial tumors are often the major differential for infarct. Often the scenario will be a patient thought originally to have an infarct, but as time goes on, and repeat scans show atypical patterns of enhancement, the neurosurgeons become involved. Both infarcts and tumors may be necrotic, with gemistocytic cells that can be difficult to reliably pigeonhole as reactive or neoplastic. The higher grade the glial tumor is the more likely it is to have a lymphocytic reaction, which would also be common adjacent to infarct. Reactive blood vessels may be mistaken on frozen sections for the complex microvascular changes of higher grade gliomas. But "pseudopalisading" (Fig. 3E.13) around necrosis makes it diagnostic of tumor (true pseudopalisades are not made up of inflammatory cells, so be careful). Well developed "glomeruloid" vascular changes are also consistent with high-grade glioma. Large, hyperchromatic, irregular, "bare" nuclei are neoplastic. They are not going to be reactive astrocytes (which have a cytoplasmic reaction in addition to nuclear changes). Fortunately, most high-grade gliomas reach a level of cellularity that puts anything reactive out of the differential, but we all know that the attempts of the neurosurgeon to stay out of the necrotic center, often put them too far out toward the edges of the tumor. And it is always possible for what you are looking at to be infarct when the neurosurgeon is adamant that he has a tumor in front of him, because occasionally you will see infarct next to tumor.

Differential Diagnosis: PML

The patient usually has a history of immunocompromise in progressive multifocal leukoencephalopathy (PML). Macrophages and perivascular lymphocytic cuffs are common to both PML (Fig. 3E.14) and subacute infarcts. The distribution on scans is usually different enough on larger wedgeshaped infarcts to make biopsy unusual, but infarcts in other white matter areas may be biopsied to differentiate them from tumor, MS, or PML. PML has bizarre astrocytes and oligodendroglial nuclear inclusions, unlike infarcts.

Differential Diagnosis: MS

Macrophages and perivascular lymphocytic cuffs are common to both multiple sclerosis (MS) (Fig. 3E.15) and subacute infarcts. The common age ranges for each rarely overlap. The usual distributions on scans are different. But every year we get one or more biopsies where the patient is outside the usual age range for MS and not immunocompromised, the locations are unusual for infarcts, and the neuroradiologist can't really tell what the process is on scans (other than probably not neoplastic). These often end up being an atypical demyelinating process, possibly tumefactive MS.

Differential Diagnosis: Abscess

Both infarcts and abscesses can have gliosis, macrophages, and reactive vessels. Infarcts have dead vessels within them, while abscesses tend to "push" the normal tissue away. Abscesses usually have more mitoses than infarcts. Neutrophils are not as common in infarcts as in abscesses (Fig. 3E.16).

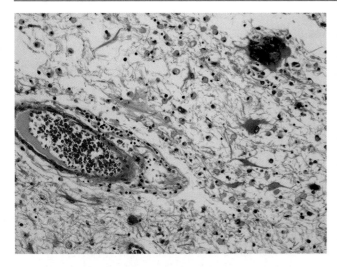

Fig. 3E.14 Histology – PML – bizarre astrocytes and numerous macrophages, with perivascular lymphocytes

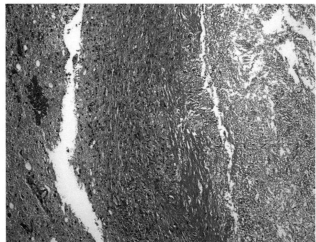

Fig. 3E.17 Histology – abscess – three zones from outside in – gliotic brain, fibrotic wall, necrotic center

Infarcts have less tendency to incite a fibrotic reaction/wall than abscesses do (Fig. 3E.17). The wall of an abscess will be apparent on scans as a ring of enhancement.

Cautions

- Red neurons are often pyramidal in shape (as opposed to gemistocytes).
- Macrophages in any significant quantities should make you think twice before calling a lesion a primary tumor.
- Don't forget infarct may be seen next to tumor, so if the surgeon insists that there is a tumor, then suggest he may be adjacent to it.

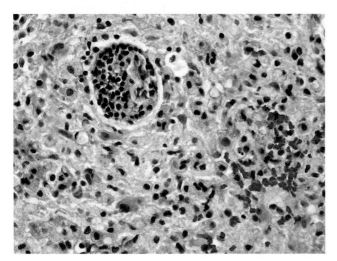

Fig. 3E.15 Histology – MS – perivascular lymphocytes, macrophages, reactive astrocytes

Bibliography

Infarct

1 Shi Y, Morgenstern N. Granular cell astrocytoma. Arch Pathol Lab Med. 2008;132(12):1946–50.
2 Agrawal A, Balpande DN, Khan A, Vagh SJ, Shukla S, Chopra S. Sickle cell crisis leading to extensive necrosis in a low-grade glioma and masquerading high-grade lesion. Pediatr Neurosurg. 2008;44(6):471–3.
3 Tanaka Y, Uematsu Y, Owai Y, Itakura T. Two cases of ring-like enhancement on MRI mimicking malignant brain tumors. Brain Tumor Pathol. 2006;23(2):107–11.
4 Lucchinetti CF, Gavrilova RH, Metz I, Parisi JE, Scheithauer BW, Weigand S, Thomsen K, Mandrekar J, Altintas A, Erickson BJ, König F, Giannini C, Lassmann H, Linbo L, Pittock SJ, Brück W. Clinical and radiographic spectrum of pathologically confirmed tumefactive multiple sclerosis. Brain 2008;131(Pt 7):1759–75
5 Iqbal M, Shah A, Wani MA, Kirmani A, Ramzan A. Cytopathology of the central nervous system. Part I. Utility of crush smear cytology in intraoperative diagnosis of central nervous system lesions. Acta Cytol. 2006;50(6):608–16.
6 Zeman D, Adam P, Kalistová H, Sobek O, Anděl J, Anděl M. Cerebrospinal fluid cytologic findings in multiple sclerosis. A comparison between patient subgroups. Acta Cytol. 2001;45(1):51–9.

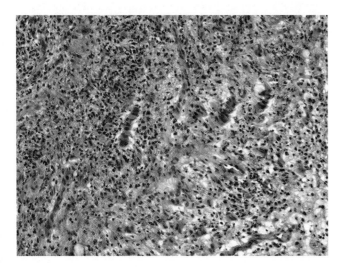

Fig. 3E.16 Histology – abscess – reactive vessels and inflammatory cells

Case 3F
A 74-Year-Old Female with Headache, Confusion and Personality Change

Cynthia T. Welsh

Clinical History

- 74-year-old female
- 2-week history of confusion, headaches, personality change
- Normal neurologic exam

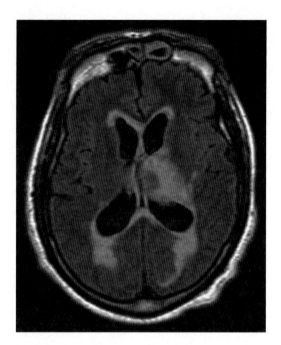

Fig. 3F.2 Axial MRI T2 FLAIR – left periventricular area dark on T2 with surrounding brighter areas demonstrating mass effect (pushing on ventricle)

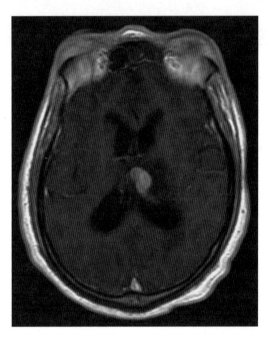

Fig. 3F.1 Axial MRI T1 postcontrast – left periventricular fairly solid contrast enhancement

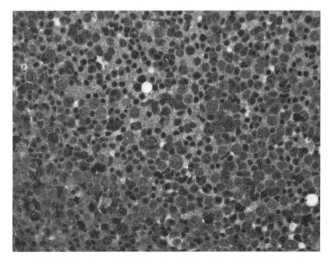

Fig. 3F.3 Touch preparation (DQ stain high magnification) – very cellular with a broad range in cell size, but predominately round nuclei in all cell sizes; nucleoli are seen in the larger nuclei

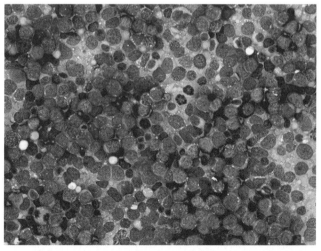

Fig. 3F.4 Touch preparation (DQ stain high magnification) – closer view of cells

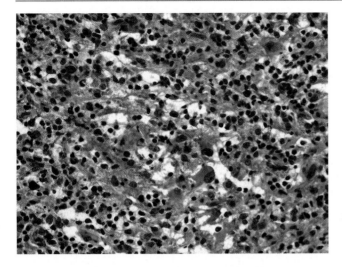

Fig. 3F.5 Frozen section (H&E stain high magnification) – astrocytes with obvious cytoplasm are sprinkled in a background of infiltrative pleomorphic cells

Fig. 3F.6 Frozen section (H&E stain low magnification) – elsewhere in the lesion, the infiltrating cells tend to coalesce cuff around vessels

What Is Your Diagnosis?

Figure Discussion

Scans

"Ring-enhancing" necrosis has a large differential which changes based on age group and immune system status. Position of the lesion as white matter centered (probably glioma) versus adjacent to ventricle (more likely PCNSL), single versus multiple lesions (could be metastatic), and the so-called open ring of MS enhancement all influence the differential. This lesion is near the ventricle and obstructing flow, causing hydrocephalus (likely a cause of the patient's symptoms). It enhances and after fluid attenuation on the FLAIR sequence shows infiltration, not just edema surrounding the main tumor mass (unlike a metastasis) (Figs. 3F.1–3F.2).

Pathology

The perivascular pattern of these cells is "cuffing" the vessels, in distinction from the nonspecific look of a glial cell "secondary structure" gravitation toward vessels, or the other patterned "pseudorosette" morphology of ependymal tumors. On the frozen section it can be difficult to tell what cell type is making up the tumor, but on the cytologic preparation the lymphoid nature of these cells is obvious, making the touch preparation invaluable. On the smears, there are large cells with little cytoplasm, large mostly round nuclei, and prominent nucleoli. The chromatin is evenly clumped (Figs. 3F.3–3F.6).

Diagnosis: Primary CNS B-Cell Lymphoma

The common age range for PCNSL, metastases, and high-grade glial lesions tends to be similar (older adult). Immunocompromise favors PCNSL, as does a location closer to ventricles, so clinical information is important. Single cell death is common in lymphomas unlike glial tumors. Perivascular cuffs of cells predominate around the periphery of the tumor, while the center consists of sheets of cells. These may have distinct cell membranes, mimicking a sheet of epithelial cells. On cytologic preparations, the single cell character will be easily seen. Almost all primary brain lymphomas are large B-cell lymphomas. They usually have large nuclei, prominent nucleoli, and little cytoplasm just like their systemic counterparts. Recognizing the lymphoid nature of the process allows you to send material to flow cytometry, and allows the neurosurgeon to stop the procedure before resection (PCNSL is not a surgical disease).

Differential Diagnosis: Metastases (Particularly Melanoma)

One metastatic lesion in particular (melanoma) has a marked tendency to single cell infiltration, which may make it more difficult to separate out from primary tumors, both glial and lymphoid, on frozen sections. You are also likely to have single cells on the cytologic preparations for both melanoma (Fig. 3F.7) and lymphoma. The nuclear characteristics will vary depending on melanoma type, ranging from spindled to large cells with large eccentric nuclei and large nucleoli (they are generally more prominent even than the ones in PCNSBL).

Differential Diagnosis: Glioma

Frozen sections can distort lymphoma nuclei infiltrating through brain and make it difficult to tell them from glial cells. Both lymphomas and gliomas may show necrosis. It may be hard in frozen sections to tell that the cells surrounding vessels (Fig. 3F.8) are glial rather than lymphoid. Smears of oligodendroglial tumors (Fig. 3F.9) can mimic lymphoma; neither have processes, both can have single cells. The nuclei in oligodendrogliomas do not generally approach the large size of the PCNSBL nuclei though. The chromatin pattern is not clumped in oligodendroglioma cells as it is in lymphoma. Necrosis in glial tumors may be pseudopalisading (unlike lymphomas) and seldom shows the single cell apoptotic pattern that is usually prominent in lymphomas.

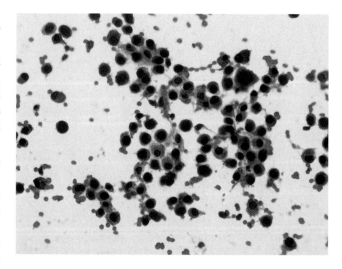

Fig. 3F.7 Smear – melanoma – large single cells with large mostly round nuclei and nucleoli

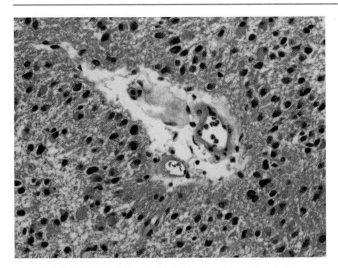

Fig. 3F.8 Histology – glioma – secondary structure of tumor cells around vessel

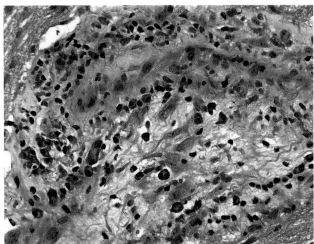

Fig. 3F.10 Histology – toxoplasmosis – no organisms are seen in this field. The vessel on the right is surrounded by lymphocytes and plasma cells

Cautions

- Primary lymphomas are infiltrative like gliomas.
- Melanomas can be somewhat infiltrative.
- Cytologic preparations (and perhaps Diff Quik stains) may make it much easier to recognize the infiltrative cell type.

Bibliography

Primary CNS B-Cell Lymphoma

1 Wu JM, Georgy MF, Burroughs FH, Weir EG, Rosenthal DL, Ali SZ. Lymphoma, leukemia, and pleiocytosis in cerebrospinal fluid: is accurate cytopathologic diagnosis possible based on morphology alone? Diagn Cytopathol. 2009;37(11):820–4.
2 Manucha V, Zhao F, Rodgers W. Atypical lymphoid cells in cerebrospinal fluid in acute Epstein Barr virus infection: a case report demonstrating a pitfall in cerebrospinal fluid cytology. Acta Cytol. 2008;52(3):334–6.
3 Iqbal M, Shah A, Wani MA, Kirmani A, Ramzan A. Cytopathology of the central nervous system. Part I. Utility of crush smear cytology in intraoperative diagnosis of central nervous system lesions. Acta Cytol. 2006;50(6):608–16.
4 Han JH, Kim JH, Yim H. Intravascular lymphomatosis of the brain. Report of a case using an intraoperative cytologic preparation. Acta Cytol. 2004;48(3):411–4
5 Roma AA, Garcia A, Avagnina A, Rescia C, Elsner B. Lymphoid and myeloid neoplasms involving cerebrospinal fluid: comparison of morphologic examination and immunophenotyping by flow cytometry. Diagn Cytopathol. 2002;27(5):271–5.
6 Nassar DL, Raab SS, Silverman JF, Kennerdell JS, Sturgis CD. Fine-needle aspiration for the diagnosis of orbital hematolymphoid lesions. Diagn Cytopathol. 2000;23(5):314–7.

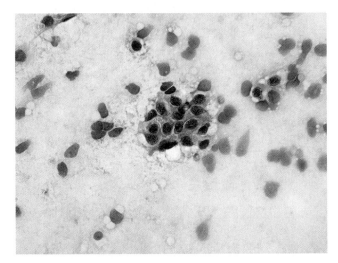

Fig. 3F.9 Smear – oligodendroglioma – small monotonous cells with a small amount of cytoplasm

Differential Diagnosis: Non-neoplastic Lymphoid Proliferations

Lymphoid infiltrates are common in many processes in brain, both neoplastic and non-neoplastic, and often form perivascular cuffs (Fig. 3F.10). Plasma cells can be an indication that the process is reactive, as can the size of the lymphoid cells which remain smaller than tumor cells.

Case 3G
A 65-Year-Old Male with Dizziness and Left Arm/Leg Weakness

Cynthia T. Welsh

Clinical History

- 65-year-old male
- Found down, "dizzy"
- Had been having left arm and leg weakness for 2 weeks
- Arteriovenous malformation in 1995; craniotomy ×2
- History: hypertension, congenital heart failure, atrial fibrillation

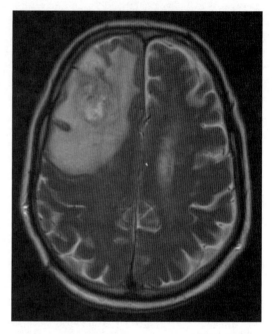

Fig. 3G.2 Axial MRI T2 – changes are seen extending all the way to the surface of the brain

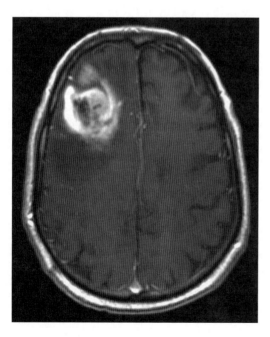

Fig. 3G.1 Axial MRI T1 postcontrast – ring-enhancing lesion in the white matter of the anterior right hemisphere

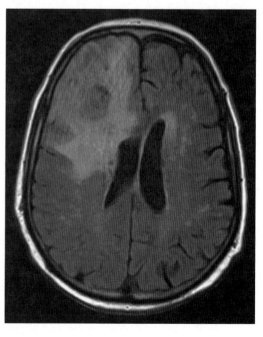

Fig. 3G.3 Axial MRI T2 FLAIR – CSF is dark, there is very little change in the signal around the central enhancing focus

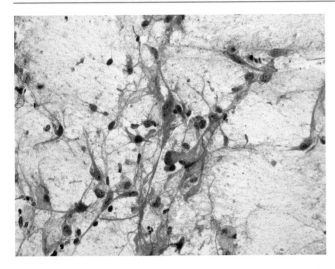

Fig. 3G.4 Smear (H&E stain high magnification) – large spindle cells with a somewhat bipolar morphology, coarse chromatin, and multiple chromocenters in addition to nucleoli

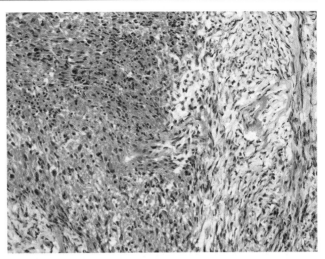

Fig. 3G.6 Frozen section (H&E stain low magnification) – areas of spindled nuclei such as seen on the smear, and adjacent more gemistocytic morphology

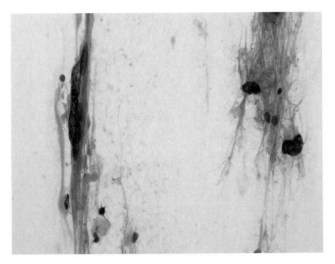

Fig. 3G.5 Smear (H&E stain high magnification) – large spindle cell (*left*) and more obvious astrocytes (*right*)

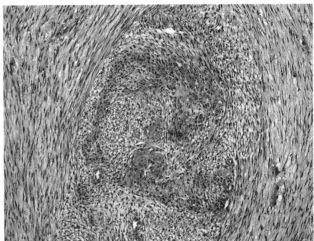

Fig. 3G.7 Frozen section (H&E stain low magnification) – spindled cells in fascicles, and cells with a rounder appearance to their morphology

What Is Your Diagnosis?

Figure Discussion

Scans

Ring-enhancing lesions which approach the brain surface may be metastatic to leptomeninges or gray–white junction with growth in both parenchymal and extra-axial directions. On the other hand, they may be gliosarcomas (Figs. 3G.1–3G.3).

Pathology

The biphasic appearance to the tumor may be explained by a tumor which is glial but has focally taken on a more spindled appearance. There are large spindle cells with a somewhat bipolar morphology, coarse chromatin, and multiple chromocenters in addition to nucleoli and cells with more obviously fibrillary astrocytic processes (finer, multiple) (Figs. 3G.4–3G.7).

Diagnosis: Gliosarcoma

Gliosarcoma is a high-grade glioma, generally glioblastoma, with the same prognosis. So you may ask, why include a separate case; why single it out? Mostly because of the confusion that it can cause for the pathologist and neurosurgeon. If you are expecting a glioblastoma and end up with ugly spindle cells instead, it shouldn't necessarily make you radically change your thinking. Somewhere in the tumor will be seen the characteristic features of glioblastoma (Figs. 3G.8 and 3G.9), although perhaps not on the material sent intraoperatively. Knowing that the tumor is intra-axial (in brain), single, with the typical scanning characteristics of a primary tumor should correlate with ugly spindle cells to make you think of gliosarcoma. This subset of GBM tends to be more often seen in temporal lobe, but can be seen elsewhere.

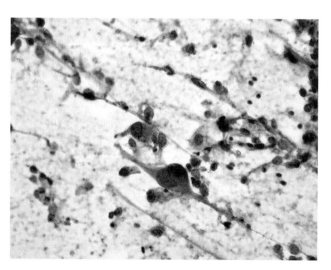

Fig. 3G.8 Smear – GBM – large pleomorphic cells with fine chromatin

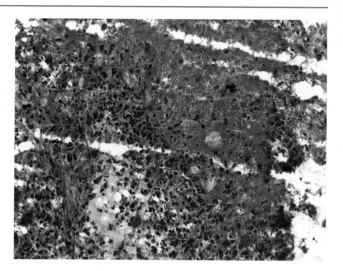

Fig. 3G.9 Histology – GBM – pleomorphic astrocytes and large scale necrosis

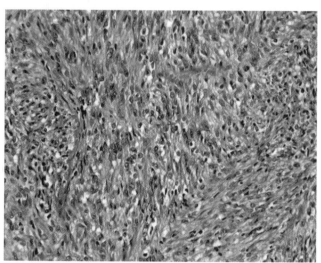

Fig. 3G.10 Histology – sarcoma – fascicles of spindle cells with mitoses

Differential Diagnosis: Primary or Metastatic Sarcoma

The major differential would include other spindle cell tumors, whether primary or metastatic in the leptomeninges, or possibly brain. Systemic sarcomas infrequently metastasize to the brain, dura, or skull. Primary high-grade tumors are most often of the malignant meningioma or hemangiopericytoma variety. Primary or metastatic dural spindle cell malignancies (Fig. 3G.10) are much less common than "sarcomatous" transformation of a glioblastoma.

Bibliography

Gliosarcoma

1   Hayashi T, Kushida Y, Kadota K, Katsuki N, Bando K, Miyai Y, Funamoto Y, Haba R. Cytopatholologic features of gliosarcoma with areas of primitive neuroepithelial differentiation of the brain in squash smears. Diagn Cytopathol. 2009;37(12):906–9.
2   Sioutopoulou DO, Kampas LI, Gerasimidou D, Valeri RM, Boukovinas I, Tsavdaridis D, Destouni CT. Diagnosis of metastatic tumors in cerebrospinal fluid samples using thin-layer cytology. Acta Cytol. 2008;52(3):304–8.
3   Shukla K, Parikh B, Shukla J, Trivedi P, Shah B. Accuracy of cytologic diagnosis of central nervous system tumours in crush preparation. Indian J Pathol Microbiol. 2006;49(4):483–6.
4   Parwani AV, Berman D, Burger PC, Ali SZ. Gliosarcoma: cytopathologic characteristics on fine-needle aspiration (FNA) and intraoperative touch imprint. Diagn Cytopathol. 2004;30(2):77–81.
5   Collaço LM, Tani E, Lindblom I, Skoog L. Stereotactic biopsy and cytological diagnosis of solid and cystic intracranial lesions. Cytopathology 2003;14(3):131–5.

Case 3H
A 39-Year-Old Male with New-Onset Seizures

Cynthia T. Welsh

Clinical History

- 39-year-old male
- New onset seizures versus anxiety attacks
- Head injury 3 years ago
- Exam: normal

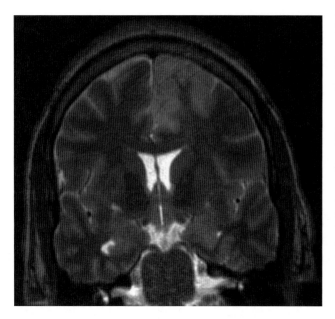

Fig. 3H.1 Coronal MRI T2 – left frontal thickening of gray matter in the anterior cerebral artery distribution with very little "mass effect"

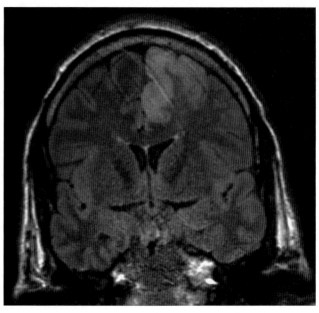

Fig. 3H.2 Coronal MRI T2 FLAIR – left frontal thickening of gray matter in the anterior cerebral artery distribution with very little "mass effect"

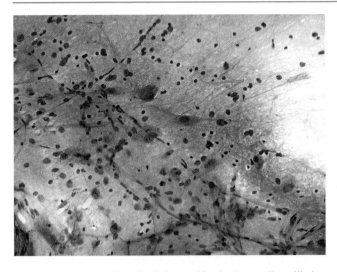

Fig. 3H.3 Smear (H&E stain high magnification) – small capillaries, background glial cells, and several neurons

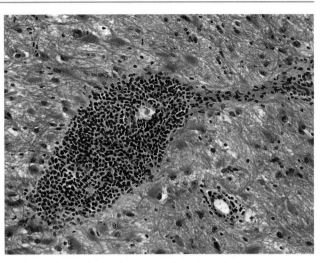

Fig. 3H.5 Frozen section (H&E stain low magnification) – gemisto-cytic astrocytes and lymphocytic "cuffing"

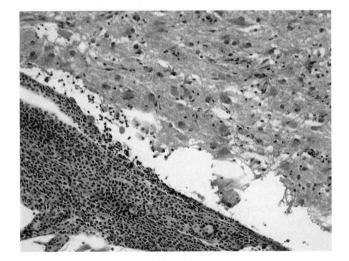

Fig. 3H.4 Frozen section (H&E stain low magnification) – gemisto-cytic astrocytes, lymphocytic infiltrate, and neurons

What Is Your Diagnosis?

Figure Discussion

Scans

This appears to be a cortical-based tumor with very little, if any, mass effect. There was no enhancement so postcontrast sequences are not shown (Figs. 3H.1–3H.2).

Pathology

Lymphocytic infiltration is not unusual in glial tumors, although not typical until higher grades (not seen here) in fibrillary (diffuse) astrocytoma. Certain low-grade tumors such as ganglioglioma have this same propensity for lymphocytic cuffing. The combination of low-grade cortical-based tumor and cuffing should lead to a search for other ganglioglioma clues such as eosinophilic granular bodies and neoplastic neurons. Two of the neurons on the smear appear to be binucleate. It is difficult to say if there are too many (we are in cortex) and they are not enormous (Figs. 3H.3–3H.5).

Diagnosis: Ganglioglioma

Realistically, the diagnosis of ganglioglioma is not one necessary at frozen section, but recognizing the neuronal aspects of the tumor can keep you from calling it high grade prematurely. Neurons (ganglion cells) are generally considered potentially neoplastic when they are too many, too large, or disorganized. Of course, that assumes you know the location of the biopsy and what appearance that tissue is supposed to have. Neurons that are binucleate are also suspect, although if you look at enough neuropathology specimens, you have undoubtedly run into binucleate neurons in "normal" brain. Knowing the clinical situation, which is most often a fairly young person with seizures and a peripheral lesion involving cortex, helps you to expect that ganglioglioma may be in the differential diagnosis. Microcysts, perivascular lymphocytic cuffing, and eosinophilic granular cytoplasmic bodies are all histologic or cytologic clues also. Features that might have made the glioma high grade, do not automatically do so when there is a ganglion cell component, so be careful not to miss these cells and overcall the tumor intraoperatively. Other CNS tumors which only occasionally have large ganglion cells as a component of the tumor include pleomorphic xanthoastrocytoma, neurocytoma, medulloblastoma, and desmoplastic infantile ganglioglioma.

Differential Diagnosis: Normal Cortex, Deep Gray Matter, Amygdala

You need to know what to expect as normal in order to decide whether to consider the neurons as possibly neoplastic. Familiarity with location of the biopsy and normal architecture at that location does not require relearning neuroanatomy. The normal rows and columns of the cortex (Fig. 3H.6) make it recognizable unless heavily overrun by tumor cells. Deep gray matter (Fig. 3H.7) can be a little more problematic unless you know the location of the biopsy. Amygdala is one area in particular where knowledge of location can be useful because it normally has many large neurons in clusters (Fig. 3H.8).

Differential Diagnosis: Neurons Trapped in Tumor

This tumor obviously involves gray matter (cortex) on scans, so neurons on the histology shouldn't be a surprise. Normal cortical neurons usually have one nucleus, are appropriately

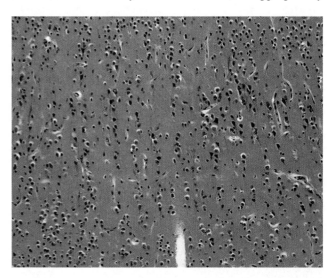

Fig. 3H.6 Histology – normal cortex with rows of small neurons (layers 2 and 4) across the top and bottom of the figure and the columns of layer 3 pyramidal neurons all pointing up toward the surface of the brain

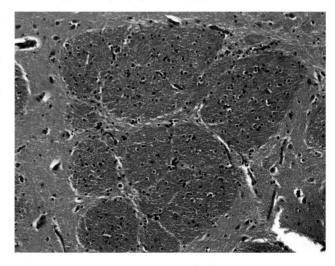

Fig. 3H.7 Histology – normal deep gray matter with clustered white matter tracts going through demonstrating chiefly an oligodendroglial population

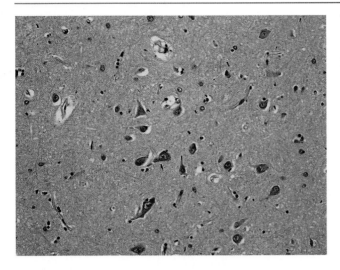

Fig. 3H.8 Histology – normal amygdala with many large, clustered neurons oriented in several different directions

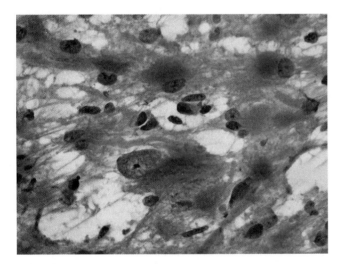

Fig. 3H.9 Histology – glioma – the ganglion cell in the center of the frame in this figure has slightly *blue* cytoplasm suggesting Nissl substance and may require immunohistochemistry to ultimately determine tumor type

sized and shaped, have cells satelliting (normal and/or neoplastic) around them and show cortical organization. The biopsy may be too small to show the organization, however. And when the lesion is in an area with many large neurons which lack the regimented organization of the cortex, such as deep gray matter and amygdala, then it can be more difficult to tell. Knowing where the biopsy is from is fundamental to knowing size, cell type, and organization parameters. Gliomas (Fig. 3H.9) can have cells with abundant cytoplasm (gemistocytic astrocytes) which sometimes must be differentiated from neurons.

Differential Diagnosis: DNET

Dysembryoplastic neuroepithelial tumor (DNET) is another tumor with ganglion cells which is typically seen in young people with seizures, and affects cortex. Multiple cortical nodules of oligodendroglial-like cells and glial processes surrounding microcysts with "floating" neurons (Fig. 3H.10) define DNET. These tumors may be completely removed.

Differential Diagnosis: SEGA

Large cells, some of which have neuronal characteristics (Fig. 3H.11) admixed with large gemistocytic appearing astrocytes are seen in subependymal giant cell astrocytoma (SEGA). Knowing the tissue is intra/periventricular in a

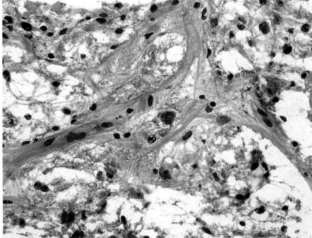

Fig. 3H.10 Histology – DNET – microcysts containing neurons

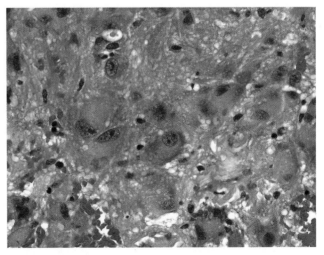

Fig. 3H.11 Histology – SEGA – large cells some with eosinophilic cytoplasm, others with what appears to be peripheral Nissl substance

patient with tuberous sclerosis (TS) goes a long way toward entering into the correct differential. Recognizing the neuronal flavor to some of these cells and calling this tumor a ganglioglioma would not actually be as problematic as calling it a gemistocytic astrocytoma (which has very negative connotations in respect to grade and prognosis).

Cautions

- All neurons are not neoplastic.
- Neoplastic ganglion type cells are often an indication of low-grade tumor.
- Ganglion cell tumors are graded differently – mitoses are not enough to make it high grade.

Bibliography

Ganglioglioma

1 Fadare O, Mariappan MR, Hileeto D, Zieske AW, Kim JH, Ocal IT. Desmoplastic Infantile Ganglioglioma: cytologic findings and differential diagnosis on aspiration material. Cytojournal. 2005;2(1):1.
2 Bleggi-Torres LF, Netto MR, Gasparetto EL, Gonçalves E Silva A, Moro M. Dysembrioplastic neuroepithelial tumor: cytological diagnosis by intraoperative smear preparation. Diagn Cytopathol. 2002;26(2):92–4.
3 Hasegawa Y, Hayabuchi Y, Namba I, Watanabe T, Kato K, Ijiri R, Tanaka Y, Sekido K, Kigasawa H, Hara M. Cytologic features of desmoplastic infantile ganglioglioma: a report of two cases. Acta Cytol. 2001;45(6):1037–42.
4 Koeller KK, Henry JM. From the archives of the AFIP: superficial gliomas: radiologic-pathologic correlation. Armed Forces Institute of Pathology. Radiographics 2001;21(6):1533–56.
5 Loesel LS. Fine needle aspiration cytology of a cerebral ganglioglioma. Report of a case. Acta Cytol. 1988;32(3):391–4.

Case 31
A 25-Year-Old Female with Headache, Nausea, Blurry Vision

Cynthia T. Welsh

Clinical History

- 25-year-old female
- Headaches, blurry vision ×2 weeks
- Intermittent nausea
- Exam:
  - Slight ptosis left upper eyelid

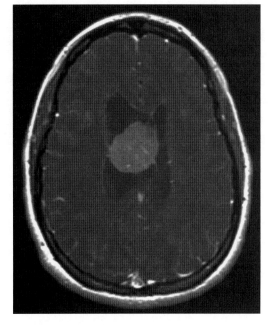

Fig. 31.2 Axial MRI T1 postcontrast – some enhancement

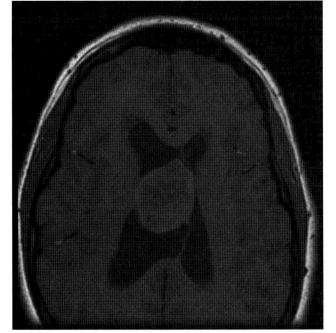

Fig. 31.1 Axial MRI T1 precontrast – intraventricular tumor attached to septum

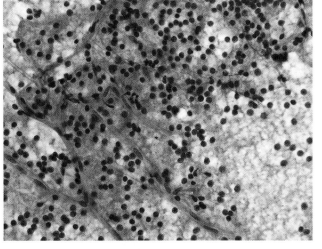

Fig. 31.3 Smear (H&E stain high magnification) – fine capillaries and numerous small round nuclei

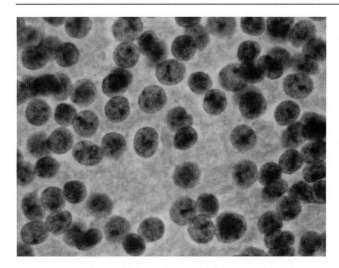

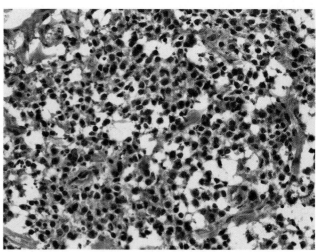

Fig. 31.4 Smear (H&E stain high magnification) – round nuclei, some condensation of chromatin at nuclear rim (rare chromocenters also), and occasional central nucleoli

Fig. 31.5 Frozen section (H&E stain high magnification) – scattered astrocytes, and many cells with frozen distortion and hyperchromaticity of nuclei, as well as a little rim of eosinophilic cytoplasm

What Is Your Diagnosis?

Figure Discussion

Scans

The septal attachment rather than an origin from the lateral wall of the ventricle or from choroid plexus narrows the differential diagnosis. Neurocytomas characteristically heterogeneously enhance. An ependymal origin would still be possible for the scan appearance (Figs. 3I.1–3I.2).

Pathology

The frozen section makes it difficult to tell the tumor cell type. The smears once again save the day by making it abundantly clear that these are small monotonous round nuclei. There are areas where the nuclei surround fine fibrillar material in neuronal rosettes. And the vessels are exclusively capillaries. There is no cytoplasmic clearing or microcalcifications (Figs. 3I.3–3I.5).

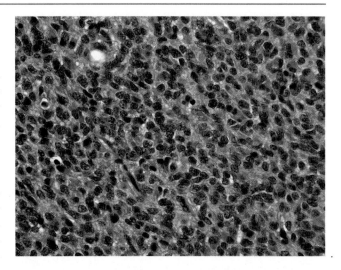

Fig. 3I.6 Histology – oligodendroglioma – cellular tumor with small nuclei and no haloes

Diagnosis: Neurocytoma

Within a ventricle, it can be possible to make neurocytoma the top ten choices for differential diagnosis when it has the distinct location within the septum. Extra-ventricular neurocytomas are more problematic. There is considerable overlap on histology between neurocytoma and oligodendroglioma. Both have haloes, microcalcifications, and a fine capillary architecture. Both can have microcysts. Neurocytoma nuclei on smears have a salt and pepper chromatin and do not generally have cytoplasm attached, but often sit in small patches of background matrix. The neuronal rosette is the distinguishing characteristic that makes a monotonous small round cell tumor recognized as a neurocytoma. These can be seen on sections but also in smears. It is important to distinguish between the well-circumscribed (removable) neurocytoma and the infiltrative oligodendroglioma (which is usually not possible to remove entirely and will eventually return, often at a higher grade).

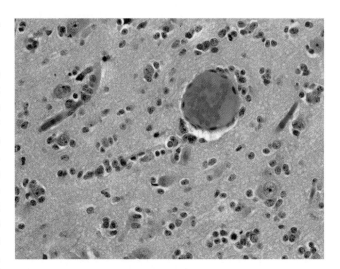

Fig. 3I.7 Histology – oligodendroglioma – tumor cells infiltrating cortex and satelliting around vessels and neurons

Differential Diagnosis: Oligodendroglioma

Central neurocytomas were misdiagnosed as oligodendrogliomas for years until they were recognized as a separate tumor category. It is probable that extra-ventricular neurocytomas continue to be misdiagnosed. They have microcalcifications, small round nuclei, and abundant capillaries, as well as enhance (though low grade) just like oligodendrogliomas. Oligodendrogliomas do not necessarily have haloes (Fig. 3I.6), and neurocytomas frequently do. In addition, however, neurocytomas have neuronal rosettes. They do not infiltrate cortex like oligodendrogliomas (Fig. 3I.7) are so inclined to do. Smears that have not had too much pressure applied may show small rims of cytoplasm attached to nuclei in oligodendrogliomas (Fig. 3I.8).

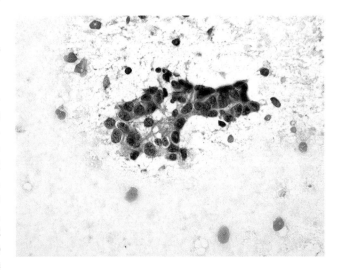

Fig. 3I.8 Smear – oligodendroglioma – single cells and small groups of small nuclei which are round to oval and have small rims of cytoplasm attached

Differential Diagnosis: Ependymoma

The differential prior to actually looking at the pathology may include ependymoma (intraventricular location!), but seldom does after microscopy of the tissue. Ependymal nuclei are more oval on cytology (Fig. 3I.9), ependymal rosettes may be seen on either cytologic preparations or on frozen section (Fig. 3I.10), and perivascular pseudorosettes are usually common. Clear cell ependymoma may resemble neurocytoma more than other subtypes because of the clear cells, microcalcifications, and sparseness of perivascular rosettes.

Differential Diagnosis: Metastatic Small Cell Carcinoma

Interestingly enough, despite the heavy vascularity of choroid plexus and the lack of blood–brain barrier there, metastases seldom appear inside ventricles preferentially. The nuclear molding, necrosis (including single cell apoptosis), and irregularity of the nuclei in a metastatic small cell carcinoma (Fig. 3I.11) would be distinct from neurocytoma especially if cytopreparations are available.

Differential Diagnosis: Subependymoma

The pattern of relatively anuclear areas in subependymoma is different than the neuronal rosette pattern of neurocytoma. Instead, in subependymoma you see round to oval nuclei in clusters with cleared areas between clusters (Fig. 3I.12). The level of cellularity varies considerably, but is less than that seen in the center of neurocytomas.

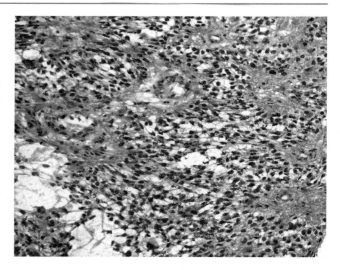

Fig. 3I.10 Histology – ependymoma – even on frozen section the relatively anuclear areas around the vessels are usually apparent if you look closely

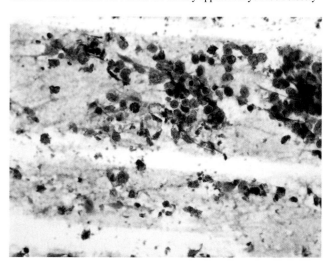

Fig. 3I.11 Histology – small cell carcinoma – necrosis, mitoses, and relatively small cells with salt and pepper chromatin and no nucleoli

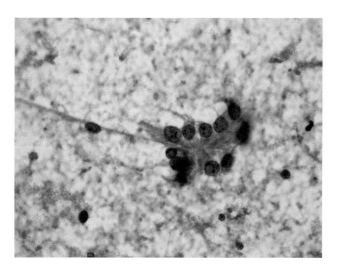

Fig. 3I.9 Smear – ependymoma – an ependymal rosette

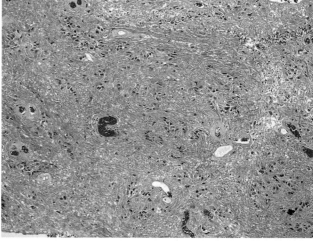

Fig. 3I.12 Histology – subependymoma – sparsely cellular tissue with clusters of nuclei embedded in the neuropil alternate with relatively anuclear areas. The vessels are somewhat hyalinized

Cautions

- All tumors with haloes are not oligodendrogliomas.
- An intraventricular tumor that looks like an oligodendroglioma probably is not one.

Bibliography

Neurocytoma

1 Klysik M, Gavito J, Boman D, Miranda RN, Hanbali F, De Las Casas LE. Intraoperative imprint cytology of central neurocytoma: the great oligodendroglioma mimicker. Diagn Cytopathol. 2010; 38(3):202–7.

2 Kobayashi TK, Bamba M, Ueda M, Nishino T, Muramatsu M, Hino A, Shima A, Echigo T, Oka H. Cytologic diagnosis of central neurocytoma in intraoperative squash preparations: a report of 2 cases. Acta Cytol. 2010;54(2):209–13.

3 Sugita Y, Tokunaga O, Morimatsu M, Abe H. Cytodiagnosis of central neurocytoma in intraoperative preparations. Acta Cytol. 2004; 48(2):194–8.

4 Ng HK. Cytologic features of central neurocytomas of the brain. A report of three cases. Acta Cytol. 1999;43(2):252–6.

5 Johnson ES, Nguyen-Ho P, Nguyen GK. Cytology of central neurocytoma in intraoperative crush preparations. A case report. Acta Cytol. 1994;38(5):764–6.

Case 3J
A 21-Month-Old Male with Developmental Regression

Cynthia T. Welsh

Clinical History

- 21-month-old male
- Decline in gross motor skills
- Exam
  - Increased muscle tone
  - Brisk reflexes
  - Ataxic even while sitting

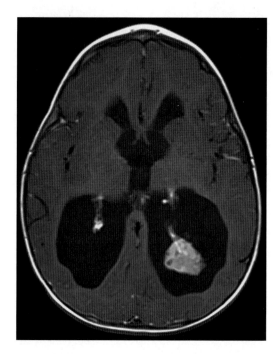

Fig. 3J.2 Axial MRI T1 postcontrast – choroid plexus vessels brighter than the mass, which does enhance

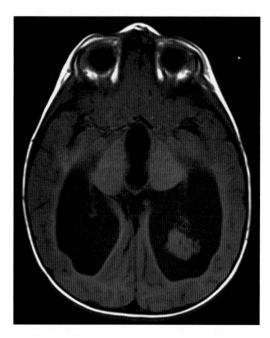

Fig. 3J.1 Axial MRI T1 precontrast – left posterior lateral ventricle mass iso-intense to brain

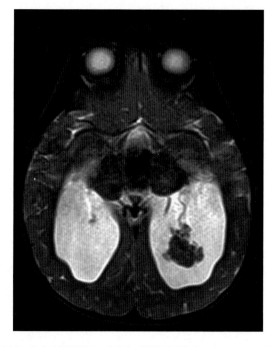

Fig. 3J.3 Axial MRI T2 – bright CSF highlights the mass which is again iso-intense to brain

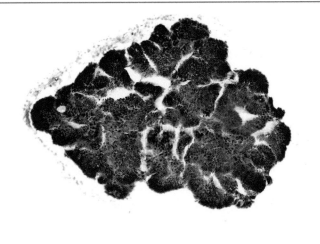

Fig. 3J.4 Smear (DQ stain, low magnification) – papillary architecture

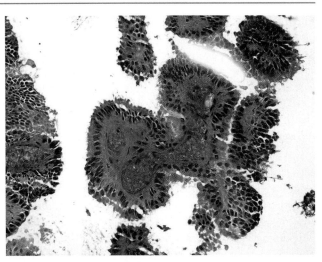

Fig. 3J.7 Frozen section (H&E stain low magnification) – papillary groups with congested vasculature

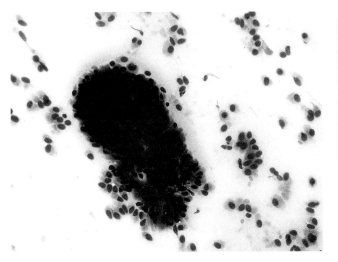

Fig. 3J.5 Smear (DQ stain, higher magnification) – one papillary group, and individual cells

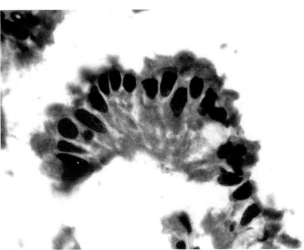

Fig. 3J.8 Frozen section (H&E stain high magnification) – round to oval nuclei with coarse chromatin, columnar cytoplasm

What Is Your Diagnosis?

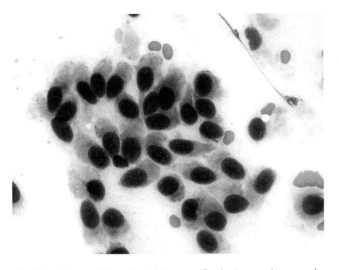

Fig. 3J.6 Smear (DQ stain, high magnification) – oval, eccentric, monotonous nuclei

Figure Discussion

Scans

The scans show an intraventricular lesion which does not enhance very brightly, in a child. It is iso-intense on both T1 and T2 sequences (Figs. 3J.1–3J.3).

Pathology

The tissue does not squash or smear well, but the papillary nature can be seen. The individual nuclei are oval and monotonous with a suggestion of eccentricity; perhaps a columnar cell pattern. The frozen sections bear this out, with a columnar covering to the papillae which is still somewhat "cobblestone" in appearance in areas, but more pseudostratified in others. This tissue fragment is not more voluminous than normal choroid plexus, but is more cellular (Figs. 3J.4–3J.8).

Diagnosis: Choroid Plexus Papilloma

Intraventricular tumors in the pediatric age group are most often ependymomas, with choroid plexus tumors being second in frequency. Ependymomas may occasionally be papillary. The most common grossly frond-like tissue from ventricle is actually choroid plexus (normal or reactive) that the neurosurgeon has encountered on the way to the tumor. Volume of tissue can often be a first indication that what you are dealing with is not normal choroid plexus so it is helpful to be familiar with how much is normal. On frozen section, the papilloma will have more cellular crowding, with loss of the normal "cobblestone" look of normal choroid plexus (Fig. 3J.9). The tissue doesn't smear well, but some individual columnar appearing cells will be seen.

The papilloma has papillary structure, but higher grade lesions often become focally more solid, cellular, and pleomorphic. Atypical papillomas have increased mitotic activity.

Differential Diagnosis: Papillary Ependymoma

Intraventricular tumors in the pediatric age group are most often conventional ependymomas, with choroid plexus tumors being second in frequency. Intracranial ependymomas may occasionally be papillary (Fig. 3J.10), and so may enter the differential diagnosis. Instead of the fibrovascular core of choroid plexus tumors, ependymomas have a delicate neuropil core. Despite the name, myxopapillary ependymomas are often NOT papillary in appearance and the perivascular pseudorosettes denote the ependymal nature of the tumors. They seldom occur in the cranium. Choroid plexus papillomas are benign tumors, although they may spread through the CSF; ependymomas require CSF analysis and scans to evaluate for drop metastases. They also require additional treatment that the papilloma does not need.

Differential Diagnosis: ELST

Knowing that the location is somewhere in temporal bone, should make an endolymphatic sac tumor (Fig. 3J.11) (ELST) enter the differential diagnosis. These tumors are papillary and can have calcifications like choroid plexus tumors, although psammoma bodies are unusual. ELST most often have only a single layer of surface cells. ELST can also have intranuclear pseudoinclusions like papillary cancer of thyroid, as well as colloid-like material. Extension of the

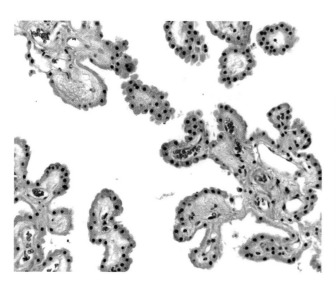

Fig. 3J.9 Histology – normal choroid plexus with a fibrovascular core and single cell layer covering the core

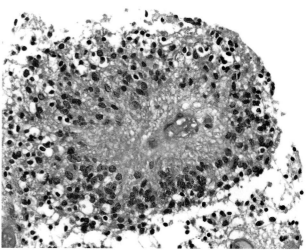

Fig. 3J.10 Histology – ependymoma – the area between the nuclei and the vessel consists of the fine processes of ependymal cells

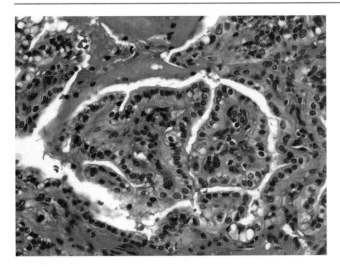

Fig. 3J.11 Histology – ELST – papillary structures with fibrovascular cores and bland cells covering the cores

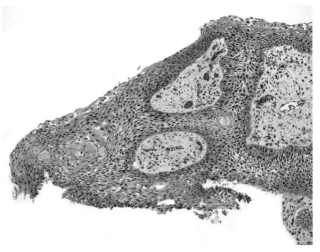

Fig. 3J.12 Histology – craniopharyngioma – papillary structure covered by squamous epithelium with loose stellate reticulum centrally and focal keratinization

ELST often results in cerebellar and further skullbase involvement. The diagnosis should trigger exclusion of von Hippel–Lindau syndrome clinically.

Differential Diagnosis: Papillary Craniopharyngioma

Papillary craniopharyngioma (Fig. 3J.12), in contrast to the more common adamantinomatous subtype, has a tendency to involve the third ventricle. It may then enter into the differential of papillary intraventricular tumors. The distinctive basal palisading of cells and intracellular bridging may usually be easily distinguished on frozen section. These have less tendency toward stellate reticulum and do not have the "wet keratin" and calcification pattern of the adamantinomatous subtype.

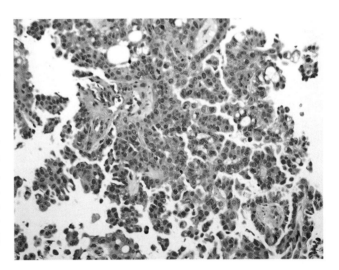

Fig. 3J.13 Histology – metastatic adenocarcinoma – papillary tumor which is mitotically active and demonstrates nucleoli

Differential Diagnosis: Papillary Metastatic Tumor

Most papillary tumors metastatic to the CNS are adenocarcinomas (Fig. 3J.13). Fortunately, few are low grade enough to seriously enter the differential with choroid plexus papilloma. They may be considered in the differential with higher grade choroid plexus neoplasms, although the choroid plexus carcinoma is seldom seen outside of childhood.

Differential Diagnosis: Papillary Meningioma

Meningiomas can occur in ventricles and they are rarely papillary, although many tend to fall apart and have a papillary type look in some areas (Fig. 3J.14). Both tumors can have psammoma bodies. The characteristic whirls and/or intranuclear pseudoinclusions will often be present somewhere within the tissue of a meningioma.

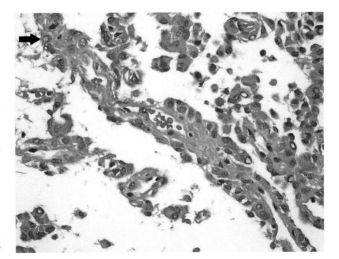

Fig. 3J.14 Histology – meningioma – intranuclear pseudoinclusions (*arrow*) help to discriminate from some of the other tumors

Cautions

Normal choroid plexus is the most common papillary tissue to be found in the ventricles.

Bibliography

Papilloma

1 Qian X, Goumnerova LC, De Girolami U, Cibas ES. Cerebrospinal fluid cytology in patients with ependymoma: a bi-institutional retrospective study. Cancer 2008;114(5):307–14.
2 Parwani AV, Stelow EB, Pambuccian SE, Burger PC, Ali SZ. Atypical teratoid/rhabdoid tumor of the brain: cytopathologic characteristics and differential diagnosis. Cancer 2005;105(2):65–70.
3 Koeller KK, Sandberg GD. From the archives of the AFIP. Cerebral intraventricular neoplasms: radiologic-pathologic correlation. Armed Forces Institute of Pathology. Radiographics 2002;22(6):1473–505.
4 Parwani AV, Fatani IY, Burger PC, Erozan YS, Ali SZ. Colloid cyst of the third ventricle: cytomorphologic features on stereotactic fine-needle aspiration. Diagn Cytopathol. 2002;27(1):27–31.
5 Otani M, Fujita K, Yokoyama A, Shimizu T, Serizawa H, Kudo M, Ebihara Y. Imprint cytologic features of intracytoplasmic lumina in ependymoma. A report of two cases. Acta Cytol. 2001;45(3):430–4.
6 Pai RR, Kini H, Rao VS, Naik R. Choroid plexus papilloma diagnosed by crush cytology. Diagn Cytopathol. 2001;25(3):165–7.
7 Murphy BA, Geisinger KR, Bergman S. Cytology of endolymphatic sac tumor. Mod Pathol. 2001;14(9):920–4.
8 Buchino JJ, Mason KG. Choroid plexus papilloma. Report of a case with cytologic differential diagnosis. Acta Cytol. 1992;36(1):95–7.

The Infratentorial Intra-axial Tumor

4

Case 4A
A 15-Year-Old Female with Headache, Nausea, and Vomiting

Cynthia T. Welsh

Clinical History

- 15-year-old female
- 4-day history headache, nausea, vomiting, ataxia, neck pain, blurry vision
- Exam:
  - Mild right nystagmus
  - Decreased right rapid alternating movements
  - Right side dysmetria

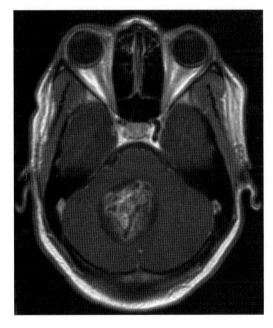

Fig. 4A.1 Axial T1 MRI postcontrast – heterogeneous enhancement, small cystic spaces

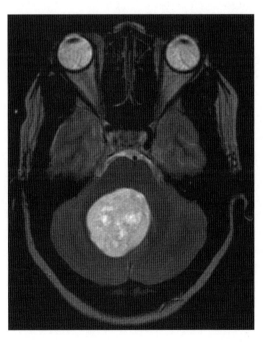

Fig. 4A.2 Axial T2 MRI – bright with fluid in cystic spaces brighter

C.T. Welsh (✉)
Department of Pathology and Laboratory Medicine,
Medical University of South Carolina, Charleston, SC 29425, USA
e-mail: welshct@musc.edu

C.T. Welsh (ed.), *Intra-Operative Neuropathology for the Non-Neuropathologist: A Case-Based Approach*,
DOI 10.1007/978-1-4419-1167-4_4, © Springer Science+Business Media, LLC 2012

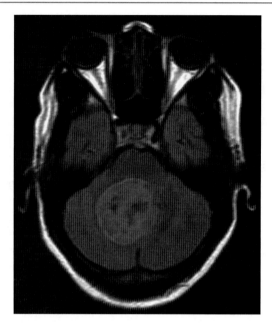

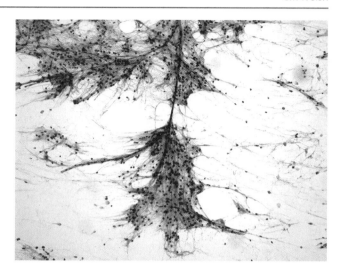

Fig. 4A.5 Smear (H&E stain low magnification) – cells "feathering" off the vessels

Fig. 4A.3 Axial T2 FLAIR MRI – tumor remains brighter than surrounding cerebellum; cyst fluid signal attenuated

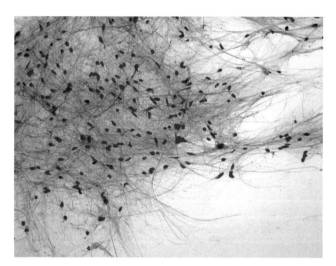

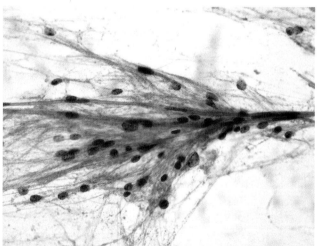

Fig. 4A.4 Smear (H&E stain high magnification) – oval nuclei, Rosenthal fibers

Fig. 4A.6 Smear (H&E stain high magnification) – closer view of cells "feathering" off the vessels

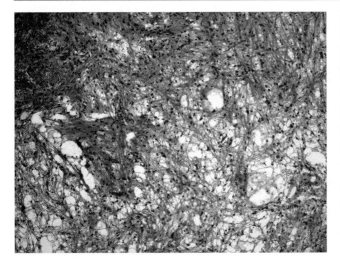

Fig. 4A.7 Frozen section (H&E stain low magnification) – Rosenthal fibers, microcysts

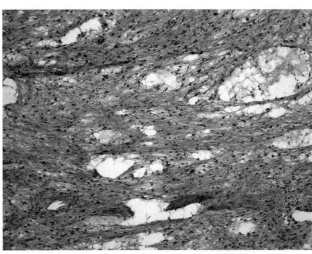

Fig. 4A.8 Frozen section (H&E stain low magnification) – enlarged, hyperchromatic nuclei

What Is Your Diagnosis?

Figure Discussion

Scans

Central cerebellar tumor, which heterogeneously enhances, is dark on T1 and bright on T2 (but not as bright on FLAIR). The cyst fluid is bright on T2 (Figs. 4A.1–4A.3).

Pathology

The tumor smears unevenly with cells clinging to vessels. The nuclei in these clinging cells tend to be at various levels. Here, Rosenthal fibers are fairly numerous and most of the cells are monotonous spindle cells, with occasional large dark nuclei. The biphasic nature of the tissue (with microcysts) is seen only on the frozen sections. The bipolar, hair-like (piloid) cells define the pilocytic astrocytoma (Figs. 4A.4–4A.8).

Diagnosis: Pilocytic Astrocytoma

Tumors in children are most commonly located in the posterior fossa (70% in the posterior fossa versus 30% above the tentorium). The most common glioma in children is the pilocytic astrocytoma (also known as juvenile pilocytic astrocytoma) of the cerebellum. The tumor also occurs in the diencephalon, optic nerves, and uncommonly spinal cord. The tumor rarely also occurs in adults. Clinically, the tumors produce symptoms appropriately related to site, such as ataxia or visual symptoms, and are often cystic; perhaps even have a "cyst with mural nodule" (Table 4A.1) on scans, especially in the cerebellum. Pilocytic astrocytomas in other sites cause an enlarged optic nerve, or spinal cord, or an exophytic lesion on the side of the medulla. They are distinct in border with surrounding tissue, enhance with contrast (unlike low-grade fibrillary astrocytomas), and often display high T_2 signal intensity. The surgeon may find a distinct plane between tumor and adjacent neuropil.

At the time of frozen, our first clue is the age of the patient, usually under 20, often under 10 years. In children, in the cerebellum, the chief diagnostic choices are pilocytic astrocytoma, medulloblastoma, and less commonly ependymoma. The pilocytic tumor smears well and cuts well. Smears show a tumor with prominent fibrillar, hair-like astrocytic processes and background, and often Rosenthal fibers and/or eosinophilic granular bodies. The cellularity and architectural arrangement of cells is abnormal on both squash preps and frozen sections. The tumor cells have elongate bipolar cytoplasm, which may be obscured on the frozen section, and variably sized nuclei. Mitoses are usually difficult to find, but finding mitoses in the presence of the other typical features does not void the diagnosis. Increased vasculature (usually hyalinized, often complex) and some limited nuclear atypia are

Table 4A.1 Cyst with mural nodule

Pilocytic astrocytoma
Hemangioblastoma
Ganglion cell tumors
Pleomorphic xanthoastrocytoma

Table 4A.2 Biphasic tumors

Pilocytic
Gliosarcoma
Schwannoma

Table 4A.3 Rosenthal fibers

Reactive gliosis (particularly around infarcts or slow growing tumors)
Pilocytic
Ganglion cell tumors
Occasionally seen in ependymoma/subependymoma

Table 4A.4 Scattered large irregular hyperchromatic nuclei

Pilocytic astrocytoma
Hemangioblastoma
Meningioma
Schwannoma

expected in this tumor, so don't fall into the trap of calling it high grade. The tumor is variably biphasic (Table 4A.2), having solid elongate patterns and microcysts. Rosenthal fibers (Table 4A.3) are found in the solid areas. The microcysts are easily dismissed as artifact if you have problems with ice crystals. The cells can be arranged in elongate fascicles and loosely around vessels. Scattered large, hyperchromatic, irregular nuclei are common, as in many low grade/benign tumors (Table 4A.4).

Differential Diagnosis: Piloid Gliosis

The same areas which tend to be home to pilocytic astrocytomas also demonstrate piloid gliosis (Fig. 4A.9) in response to injury. Reactive, gliotic, and inflammatory processes can superficially resemble a low-grade astrocytoma. For example, the gliotic zone around an abscess or metastasis, and gliosis adjacent to a craniopharyngioma or hemangioblastoma, can have prominent piloid processes, nuclear prominence, and Rosenthal fibers that can be very confusing. The MRI appearance and other clinical information can help avoid pitfalls. In the frozen section and squash preparation, the uniform cell density and foci of inflammation (if present) can help guide one toward a reactive process. If you find you have more Rosenthal fibers than cells, you should think of gliosis before tumor.

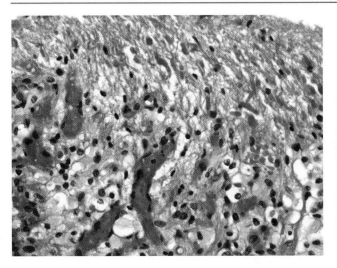

Fig. 4A.9 Histology – piloid gliosis – numerous Rosenthal fibers with scarcely any increase in cellularity adjacent to hemangioblastoma

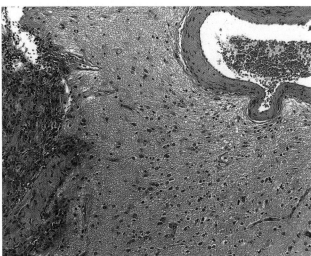

Fig. 4A.10 Histology – AVM – large vessels embedded in gliotic cerebellar white matter

Differential Diagnosis: Vascular Malformation

Pilocytic astrocytomas are very vascular, sometimes to the point where some areas within the tumor appear to be a vascular malformation. This is one of the reasons that the notion about whether the entity of an angioglioma exists has been discussed off and on for some time in the literature. The piloid gliosis that a vascular malformation (Fig. 4A.10) in the cerebellum incites would only add to the confusion. The pilocytic astrocytoma enhances on scans, whereas gliosis does not, so familiarity with the scans can be very helpful in your differential diagnosis.

Differential Diagnosis: Fibrillary Astrocytoma

Low-grade tumors on frozen section can sometimes be very difficult to separate from each other. The smears may be incredibly helpful in discriminating cell types. Pilocytic astrocytes have much more spindled (elongate) nuclei and bipolar processes as opposed to the more stellate processes of fibrillary astrocytes, although there is always some overlap (Fig. 4A.11) as seen in this fibrillary astrocytoma. Rosenthal fibers are not a characteristic finding in fibrillary astrocytomas.

Differential Diagnosis: Ependymoma

Many of the areas where pilocytic tumors are common are near ventricles. It may be possible on scans to demonstrate location, but not always. Once you have the slides, you will

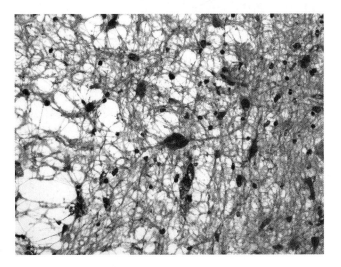

Fig. 4A.11 Histology – diffuse astrocytoma – edematous section with extensive ice crystal artifact demonstrating the bipolar appearance fibrillary astrocytes can have

find the ependymoma to be much more cellular on sections, with perivascular pseudorosettes. On smears, ependymomas have processes (Fig. 4A.12) like pilocytic astrocytomas, but the processes have a different relationship with vessels, and you may have actual ependymal rosettes on smears (Fig. 4A.13) or sections. Ependymal nuclei are oval compared to the more elongate (spindle) nuclei of pilocytic astrocytoma. In the cerebellum, differentiation between the two tumors will not be as critical as it can be in the spinal cord. Cord tumors which are ependymal will generally be removed entirely (unlike cord pilocytics) as this will generally lead to the best long-term outcome.

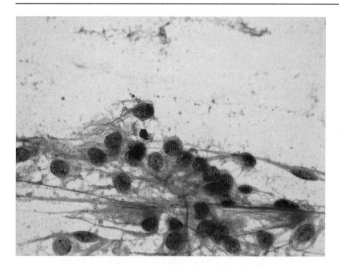

Fig. 4A.12 Smear – ependymoma – long thin processes which are somewhat similar to piloid cell processes

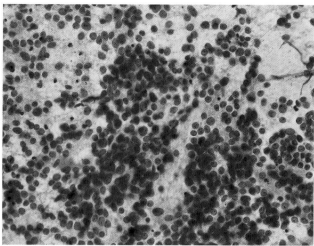

Fig. 4A.14 Smear – medulloblastoma – nuclei ranging from round to oval to baby carrot shaped with fine chromatin and very small nucleoli/chromocenters and single cell death

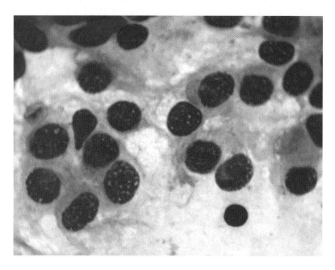

Fig. 4A.13 Smear – ependymoma – ependymal rosettes

Differential Diagnosis: Medulloblastoma

Posterior fossa tumors in children outside the ventricle are usually either pilocytic or medulloblastoma. Medulloblastomas tend to be more solid on scans. ADC mapping if available on MRI readily distinguishes between the two tumors. Smears of medulloblastoma show no processes, may show neuronal type rosettes, and have baby carrot shaped nuclei (Fig. 4A.14). Frozen sections show a very cellular tumor. Both preparations have numerous mitoses and dying single cells. More widespread necrosis may also be present.

Cautions

- Rosenthal fibers are seen in piloid gliosis as well as piloid tumors.
- Higher grade features do not negate the diagnosis of pilocytic astrocytoma and do not make it high grade.
- Pilocytic astrocytomas always enhance.

Bibliography

Pilocytic Astrocytoma

1. Ghosal N, Hegde AS, Murthy G, Furtado SV. Smear preparation of intracranial lesions: a retrospective study of 306 cases. Diagn Cytopathol. 2011;39(8):582–92.
2. Takei H, Powell SZ. Rosenthal fiber-rich glioblastoma: a case report. Clin Neuropathol. 2009;28(3):168–72.
3. Kim SH, Kim TS. Squash smear findings of eosinophilic granular bodies in pilocytic astrocytoma. Acta Cytol. 2005;49(1):112–4.
4. Browne TJ, Goumnerova LC, De Girolami U, Cibas ES. Cytologic features of pilocytic astrocytoma in cerebrospinal fluid specimens. Acta Cytol. 2004;48(1):3–8.
5. Hajdu SI. Pilocytic astrocytoma. Acta Cytol. 2004;48(1):1–2.
6. Koeller KK, Rushing EJ. From the archives of the AFIP: pilocytic astrocytoma: radiologic-pathologic correlation. Radiographics 2004; 24(6):1693–708.
7. Teo JG, Ng HK. Cytodiagnosis of pilocytic astrocytoma in smear preparations. Acta Cytol. 1998;42(3):673–8.

Case 4B
A 12-Year-Old Male with Headache, Irritability, and Vertigo

M. Timothy Smith

Clinical History

- 12-year-old boy
- Irritability, vertigo, and headaches
- Exam
  - Balance problems

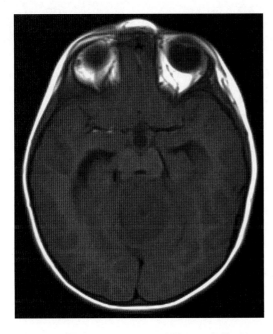

Fig. 4B.1   Axial MRI T1 precontrast – midline cerebellar tumor which is not in the fourth ventricle, but is compressing instead

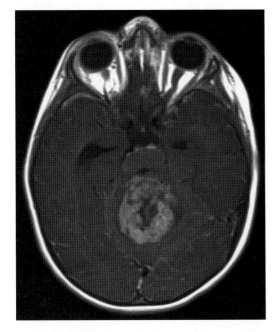

Fig. 4B.2   Axial MRI T1 postcontrast – midline cerebellar tumor with heterogeneous enhancement

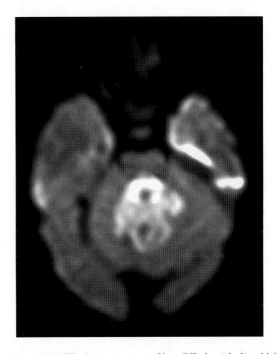

Fig. 4B.3   Axial diffusion – two areas of low diffusion (*dark*), which are likely cysts, otherwise higher diffusion than surrounding cerebellum

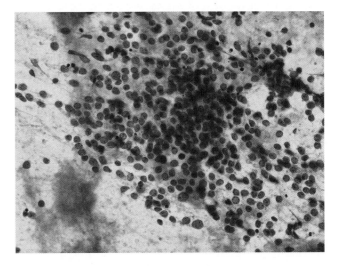

Fig. 4B.4   Smear (H&E stain high magnification) – generally small round to oval nuclei, but some nuclei with one end pointed ("baby carrot-like"); cells not clinging to vessels; pink fibrillary material with some suggestion of imperfect rings of cells around some of it

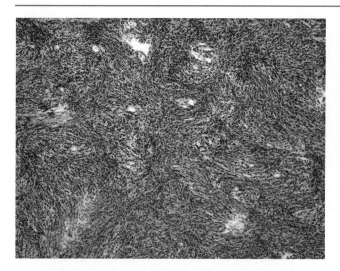

Fig. 4B.5 Frozen section (H&E stain low magnification) – cords (*rows*) of small cells

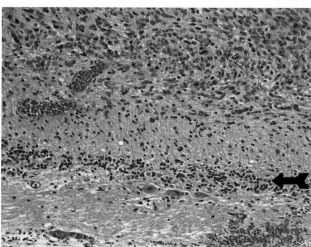

Fig. 4B.7 Frozen section (H&E stain low magnification) – tumor (*top*) near somewhat damaged cerebellum with molecular layer, Purkinje cells, and the internal granular cell layer (arrow)

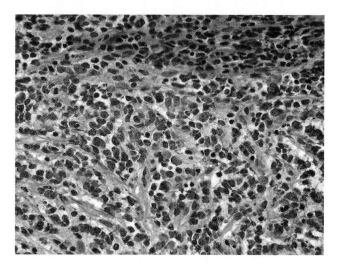

Fig. 4B.6 Frozen section (H&E stain high magnification) – a closer view with a more nested look of pleomorphic cells displaying little cytoplasm

What Is Your Diagnosis?

Figure Discussion

Scans

Midline cerebellar tumor outside the ventricle (probably not ependymal) with high diffusion compared to the rest of the brain (probably not pilocytic). That leaves medulloblastoma or atypical teratoid–rhabdoid tumor (ATRT) as the major players (Figs. 4B.1–4B.3).

Pathology

The smear shows many nuclei, most with no attached cytoplasm. There are nuclei forming incomplete rings around neuropil, and detached fragments of stroma also. The nuclei are round to oval with occasional baby carrot shapes (blunt on both ends, one end smaller than the other) and occasional tiny nucleoli. Sections show rows (single filing) of cells at low power and large nuclei with little cytoplasm and single cell death (Figs. 4B.4–4B.6). The tumor is obviously in cerebellum in Fig. 4B.7. The nuclei and rosettes in this location are consistent with medulloblastoma.

Table 4B.1 Small cell neoplasms

Medulloblastoma
PNETs (ependymoblastoma, cerebral neuroblastoma)
Small cell metastases
Lymphoma
Small cell glioblastoma
Pineoblastoma
Germinoma
Rhabdomyosarcoma, Ewing sarcoma
Esthesioneuroblastoma, SNUC (sinonasal undifferentiated carcinoma)

Table 4B.2 Neoplastic rosette types

Tumors	Rosettes
Medulloblastomas	Imperfect Homer Wright rosettes
Neuroblastomas of the adrenal	Better Homer Wright rosettes
Retinoblastomas	Flexner–Wintersteiner (true) rosettes
Ependymomas	Perivascular pseudorosettes and occasionally true rosettes

Diagnosis: Medulloblastoma

In children, most tumors are infratentorial, and the differential depends on whether the tumor is in the ventricle (think ependymoma) or not (pilocytic astrocytoma or medulloblastoma), and how cellular the lesion is which may be determined by diffusion and ADC mapping. Medulloblastoma is the name for a cerebellar tumor that can show both glial and neuronal differentiation. It is a "small blue cell tumor" (Table 4B.1) that occurs in the cerebellum as the second most common brain tumor in children. It usually affects boys, occurring less commonly in adults. It is the most common member of the CNS primitive neuroectodermal tumors (PNETs). Other members are pineoblastoma, supratentorial PNET, and ependymoblastoma. There is an association with the p53 germline mutations, and LiFraumeni and Gorlin syndromes. Clinical symptoms include cerebellar signs such as ataxia, gaze palsies, and nystagmus. MRI shows a contrast enhancing mass in the cerebellar vermis in children or the lateral cerebellar hemisphere in adults. T1-weighted images show a hypodense mass compressing or invading the fourth ventricle. MRI can identify CSF downstream "drop" metastases.

The surgeon sees the tumor as a pink mass in the cerebellum or as a white frosting-like area if the tumor invades the subarachnoid space. Hemorrhage and cystic degeneration are common findings. The tumor is soft, contributing to good smears, and frozen sections. Both smears and sections show a small cell tumor forming variably sized sheets separated by blood vessels or fibrovascular septations. In squash preparations, the cells separate from the thin blood vessels. Fibrillary background is minimal in medulloblastomas although fine fluffy cytoplasmic material may be seen between nuclei. Nuclei are oval, oblong, or baby carrot shaped with even, soft chromatin punctuated by randomly placed nucleoli (not the regularly placed nucleoli of lymphomas). Frozen sections show a tumor composed of small cells arranged back-to-back with nuclear molding and little cytoplasm. Tumor cells form imperfect irregular neuroblastic rosettes, not well-defined Homer Wright rosettes (Table 4B.2).

Mitoses and apoptotic cells are everywhere. Many tumors display amorphous sheets with a few random cells showing neuronal differentiation, but more show islands of larger cells showing glial differentiation (i.e., having pink fibrillar processes). Rare tumors have a pattern of rows and ribbons in fibrous stroma or in cerebellar white matter. The desmoplastic medulloblastoma is characterized by nodular reticulin-free areas and often linear patterns of tumor cells. The large cell medulloblastoma is composed of cells larger than usual that resemble a large cell lymphoma. Anaplastic medulloblastoma is quite pleomorphic and may resemble the ATRT; differentiation between the two can be achieved on permanent sections. Very rare medulloblastomas have rhabdomyoblastic strap cells or melanin. These last two elements if present can be confirmed on permanent sections. Intraoperative diagnosis is often "small round blue cell tumor, favor medulloblastoma."

Differential Diagnosis: Normal Cerebellum

The internal granular cell layer (Fig. 4B.8) has been mistaken for all sorts of things over the years at frozen section. Cytologic preparations can make it easier to recognize the

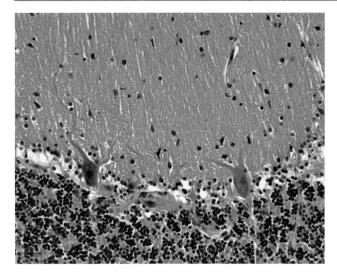

Fig. 4B.8 Histology – normal cerebellum – molecular layer at the top, small internal granular cell layer neurons across the bottom, scattered large Purkinje cells in between

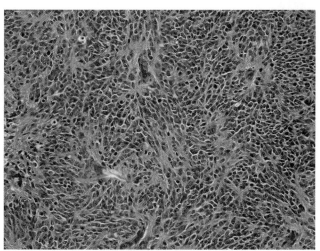

Fig. 4B.9 Histology – ependymoma – freezing the tissue makes it more difficult to see the perivascular pseudorosettes in this cellular tumor

fact that the cells you are looking at are not lymphoid (reactive or neoplastic) nuclei, and they are not some other tumor either. The nuclei are fairly monotonous and too small to be neoplastic. There are probably no (or few) mitoses and little to no apoptosis/karyorrhexis in the normal internal granular cell layer. Purkinje cells and some astrocytes will be interspersed. The normal internal granular cell layer has open spaces very much like neuronal rosettes.

Differential Diagnosis: Ependymoma

Cellular cerebellar tumors in children are generally ependymal if intraventricular, and may be medulloblastoma if intraparenchymal. Both tend to be central and it may not be easy to discriminate location on scans. Unlike the third posterior fossa tumor common in children (pilocytic astrocytoma), ependymal tumors and medulloblastomas are quite cellular. They bear many similarities on frozen sections (Fig. 4B.9) and smears (Fig. 4B.10). Usually ependymomas are less mitotically active and less necrotic, but not always. They do not have a particular propensity for single cell death. The nuclei are oval and do not have the baby carrot shape seen in medulloblastoma. Recognition of the perivascular pseudorosettes clinches the diagnosis.

Differential Diagnosis: Pineoblastoma

Medulloblastoma and pineoblastoma (Fig. 4B.11) are very similar in appearance. Some prefer to lump all these small cell tumors together. Chiefly, the decision of which tumor

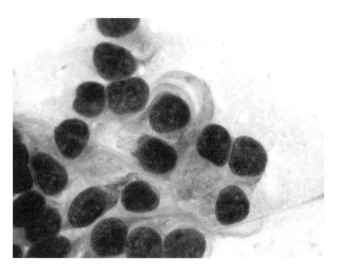

Fig. 4B.10 Smear – ependymoma – ependymal rosettes can be difficult to differentiate from neuronal rosettes

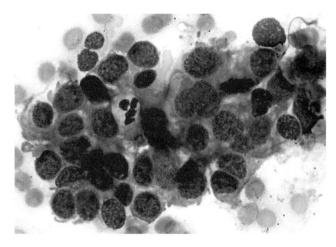

Fig. 4B.11 Smear – pineoblastoma – round to oval nuclei, small nucleoli, and a thin rim of cytoplasm

you are dealing with is made based on location, so the diagnosis is "small round blue cell tumor, defer," favoring one or the other intraoperatively.

Differential Diagnosis: PNET

A supratentorial location to the tumor which looks very similar to a medulloblastoma under the microscope should lead you to consider PNET (Fig. 4B.12) as your top contender in the differential. Intraoperatively you can once again leave the diagnosis at "small round blue cell tumor, defer."

Differential Diagnosis: Atypical Teratoid/Rhabdoid Tumor

One tumor that it is very important to eventually differentiate from medulloblastoma is the ATRT. The treatment is very different. This differentiation does not currently have to be done intraoperatively, fortunately. It can be difficult to discriminate between the two, although it may be possible to see the dense round cytoplasmic bodies (Fig. 4B.13) and eccentric nuclei (Fig. 4B.14). The atypical teratoid rhabdoid tumor is a primitive large cell medulloblastoma-like tumor with divergent differentiation identified by scattered larger keratin, EMA, and actin positive cells. Most are INI 1 negative. Diagnosis of this entity must usually wait for permanent sections and immunohistochemistry.

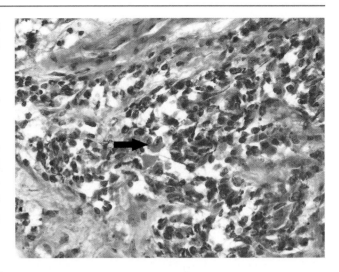

Fig. 4B.13 Histology – ATRT – the dense cytoplasmic bodies (*arrow*) are difficult to recognize on frozen section

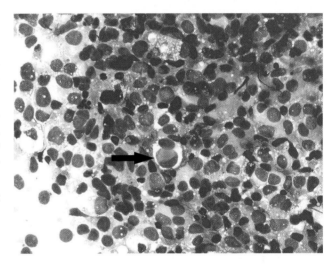

Fig. 4B.14 Smear – ATRT – the eccentricity of cytoplasm (*arrow*) in some of these cells is a clue

Differential Diagnosis: Other Small Round Blue Cell Tumors

Lymphoma and leukemias can affect the leptomeninges and dura from systemic sources at any age. Ewing's sarcoma and neuroblastoma can metastasize to skull.

Cautions

- Internal granular cells need to be distinguished from lymphocytes and tumor cells.
- Medulloblastomas cause drop metastases requiring CSF analysis.

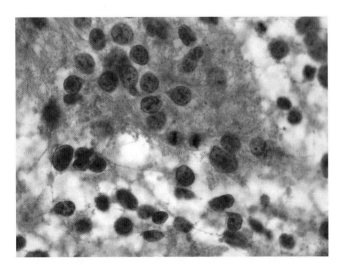

Fig. 4B.12 Smear – PNET – round to oval nuclei with multiple small chromocenters, nuclear membrane accentuation, mitoses, and neuronal rosette

Bibliography

Medulloblastoma

1. Mehta RI, Cutler AR, Lasky JL 3rd, Yong WH, Lerner JT, Hirota BK, Salamon N, Mathern GW, Vinters HV. "Primary" leptomeningeal medulloblastoma. Hum Pathol. 2009;40(11):1661–5.
2. Takei H, Dauser RC, Adesina AM. Cytomorphologic characteristics, differential diagnosis and utility during intraoperative consultation for medulloblastoma. Acta Cytol. 2007;51(2):183–92.
3. Riazmontazer N, Daneshbod Y. Cytology of desmoplastic medulloblastoma in imprint smears: a report of 2 cases. Acta Cytol. 2006; 50(1):97–100.
4. Parwani AV, Stelow EB, Pambuccian SE, Burger PC, Ali SZ. Atypical teratoid/rhabdoid tumor of the brain: cytopathologic characteristics and differential diagnosis. Cancer 2005;105(2): 65–70.
5. Raisanen J, Hatanpaa KJ, Mickey BE, White CL 3rd. Atypical teratoid/rhabdoid tumor: cytology and differential diagnosis in adults. Diagn Cytopathol. 2004;31(1):60–3.
6. Koeller KK, Rushing EJ. From the archives of the AFIP: medulloblastoma: a comprehensive review with radiologic-pathologic correlation. Radiographics 2003;23(6):1613–37.
7. Kumar PV, Hosseinzadeh M, Bedayat GR. Cytologic findings of medulloblastoma in crush smears. Acta Cytol. 2001;45(4): 542–6.
8. New KC, Bulsara KR, Dodd LG, Cummings TJ. Fine-needle aspiration diagnosis of medulloblastoma metastatic to the pelvis. Diagn Cytopathol. 2001;24(5):361–3.
9. Otani M, Fujita K, Yokoyama A, Shimizu T, Serizawa H, Kudo M, Ebihara Y. Imprint cytologic features of intracytoplasmic lumina in ependymoma. A report of two cases. Acta Cytol. 2001;45(3): 430–4.
10. Lu L, Wilkinson EJ, Yachnis AT. CSF cytology of atypical teratoid/rhabdoid tumor of the brain in a two-year-old girl: a case report. Diagn Cytopathol. 2000;23(5):329–32.

Case 4C
A 12-Year-Old Female with Headache, Nausea/Vomiting, and Vertigo

Cynthia T. Welsh

Clinical History

- 12-year-old female
- Headaches, vertigo, nausea/vomiting × months

- Exam:
  - Normal

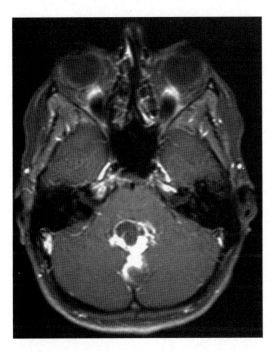

Fig. 4C.1 Axial MRI T1 postcontrast – midline cerebellar lesion with heterogeneous contrast enhancement

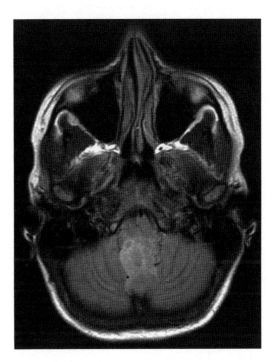

Fig. 4C.3 Axial MRI T2 FLAIR – midline cerebellar lesion

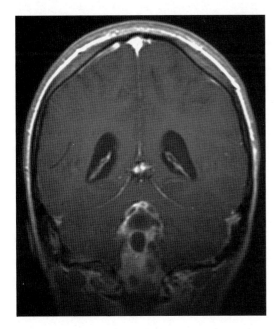

Fig. 4C.2 Coronal MRI T1 postcontrast – heterogeneous enhancement, cystic spaces, and compression of the ventricle

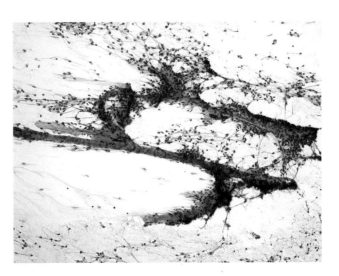

Fig. 4C.4 Smear (H&E stain low magnification) – cells clinging to vessel with cytoplasm between vessel and nucleus

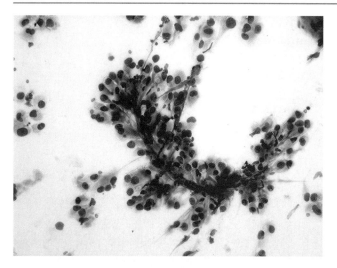

Fig. 4C.5 Smear (DQ stain high magnification) – cells clinging to vessel with cytoplasm between vessel and nucleus; round to oval nucleus

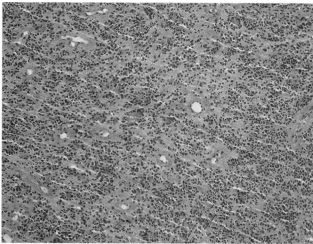

Fig. 4C.7 Frozen section (H&E stain low magnification) – perivascular areas with relatively few nuclei, and rings of cells

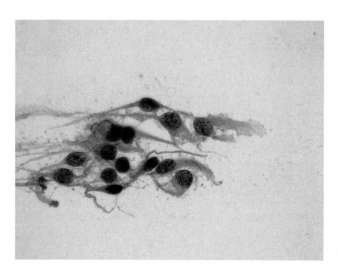

Fig. 4C.6 Smear (H&E stain high magnification) – fairly fine chromatin, chromocenters, round to oval nuclei, intracytoplasmic vacuole, and cytoplasmic processes

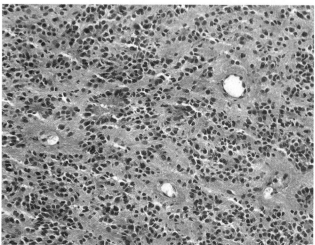

Fig. 4C.8 Frozen section (H&E stain high magnification) – perivascular areas with relatively few nuclei, and rings of cells with a suggestion of some structure at the center other than blood vessel

What Is Your Diagnosis?

Figure Discussion

Scans

It frequently requires several different views in order to determine tumor location in relationship to the ventricle. This is a midline cerebellar lesion with heterogeneous contrast enhancement and cysts, but you can't really tell if it is in the ventricle or not (Figs. 4C.1–4C.3).

Pathology

Smears showing round to oval nuclei with tiny chromocenters/nucleoli, long thin processes, and a tendency for the nuclei on cells attached to vessels to be at the end away from the vessel. Tissue sections showing not only the perivascular pseudorosettes, but also true rosettes (structures other than vessels in the center, which are only occasionally seen in ependymomas). Perivascular pseudorosettes are not exclusive to ependymomas, but in this setting are consistent with that diagnosis (Figs. 4C.4–4C.8).

Diagnosis: Ependymoma

Most intracranial ependymomas will be within the ventricular system, although occasionally one develops from the seams of ependymal cells left behind in the brain when the horns of the ventricles modify themselves during development. Patients with intracranial ependymomas are most often children (most in the fourth ventricle) or young adults. Spinal ependymomas are much more common than spinal astrocytomas and are almost exclusively seen in adults. Ependymomas are usually well circumscribed with varying contrast enhancement. Most ependymomas are only moderately cellular with a fairly monotonous population of small oval nuclei with salt and pepper chromatin and processes that extend out from vessels. The nuclei tend to be out at the ends of the cells away from the vessel (unlike astrocytic tumors where the nuclei vary in depth along the process). This creates the perivascular pseudorosette (Table 4C.1) characteristic of ependymomas, which can also be seen in other tumors, most commonly pituitary adenomas (Fig. 4C.9) which have rounder nuclei and a sellar region location of course. Usually there are few mitoses and no complex microvascular change. Some of the very large tumors seen in very young children seem to have grown as fast as their hosts, and outgrown their blood supply, leading to large-scale necrosis. Occasional cases will have ependymal rosettes and canals (Table 4C.2), which histologically resemble Flexner–Wintersteiner retinoblastoma rosettes. These can also be seen in other tumors. MRI can identify CSF downstream "drop" metastases. Spinal cord ependymomas particularly need to be intraoperatively differentiated from other tumors so that a gross total resection can be attempted, so it does help to recognize the pseudorosettes.

Table 4C.1 Perivascular pseudorosettes

Ependymoma
Pituitary adenoma
Astroblastoma
Rosette-forming glioneuronal tumor of the fourth ventricle
Papillary tumor of the pineal region
Angiocentric glioma

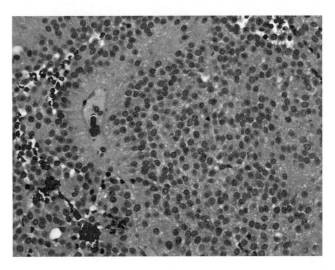

Fig. 4C.9 Histology – pituitary adenoma – monotonous round nuclei standing out away from the vessel wall

Table 4C.2 Rosettes with a nonvascular central opening

Ependymoma
Retinoblastoma
Ependymoblastoma
Embryonal tumor with abundant neuropil and true rosettes
Medulloepithelioma
Papillary tumor of the pineal region

Differential Diagnosis: Medulloblastoma

Highly cellular tumors in pediatric posterior fossa are usually either medulloblastoma in the cerebellum or ependymoma in the ventricle. Neuronal rosettes, when present, even if poorly formed (Fig. 4C.10) and lack of perivascular pseudorosettes help to discriminate between these two cellular tumors of childhood. Generally, the medulloblastoma is more cellular, more pleomorphic, more mitotically active, and has more necrosis (including single cell apoptosis). Either may have a glial appearance in areas. The medulloblastoma has ganglion cell differentiation at times.

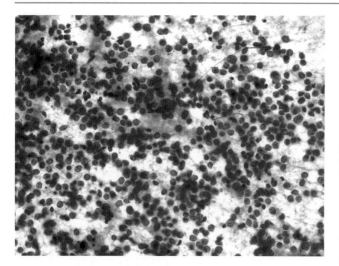

Fig. 4C.10 Smear – medulloblastoma – no processes, very little cytoplasm associated with small round to oval nuclei, and no relationship to vessels

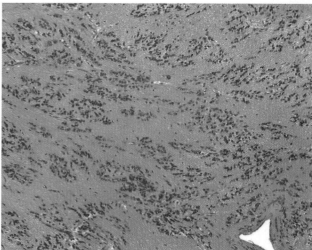

Fig. 4C.11 Histology – subependymoma – clusters of nuclei alternate with areas having a paucity of nuclei

Differential Diagnosis: Subependymoma

Relatively anuclear areas with a neuropil background exist in both of these tumors. Nuclei tend to stand out from vessels in ependymomas (perivascular pseudorosettes), while the nuclei instead cluster in subependymoma (Fig. 4C.11). There are occasions, particularly in the fourth ventricle, where both patterns exist in the same tumor, in which case it is considered an ependymoma for prognostic purposes. Otherwise this is a benign, often incidental tumor, and should not be mistaken for other tumors.

Differential Diagnosis: Glioma

Pilocytic astrocytomas in the cerebellum occur in the pediatric age group as do ependymomas. The differential should be narrowed down by MRI and ADC mapping which can separate these two tumors. If only CT has been done, then it may not be clear until you see the slides. The pilocytic astrocytoma is much less cellular and the nuclei are more spindled. If the processes are attached to a vessel wall, then the nuclei are at varying levels along those processes (Fig. 4C.12), unlike the ependymoma where they all stand out away from the vessel. Rosenthal fibers are typical of pilocytic astrocytomas, and the cerebellar tumors tend to have oligodendroglial-like areas.

Oligodendrogliomas (Fig. 4C.13) and the clear cell variant of ependymoma have many similarities. The clear cell variant has more tendency than other types to occur outside the ventricles. It has a capillary network, clear cells, and microcalcifications like oligodendrogliomas. The perivascular rosettes of ependymomas may be few and far between, requiring extensive sampling. The nuclei in oligodendrogliomas are more round than the oval ependymal nuclei.

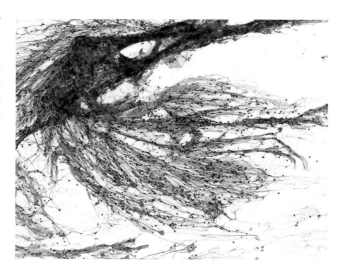

Fig. 4C.12 Smear – pilocytic astrocytoma – the cells "feather" off the vessel with the nuclei being at multiple levels along the processes

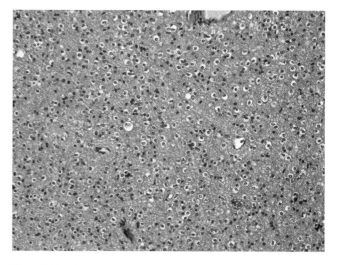

Fig. 4C.13 Histology – oligodendroglioma – haloes around mostly small round nuclei

Differential Diagnosis: Neurocytoma

The clear cell variant of ependymoma, in particular, may be similar in morphology to neurocytoma, with "haloes" and microcalcifications. Neurocytomas and ependymomas both tend to be more frequent in ventricles, but either can be extra-ventricular, (especially the clear cell variant of ependymoma). The spaces relatively devoid of nuclei in a neurocytoma do not tend to be around vessels but are instead of the neuronal rosette variety (Fig. 4C.14). Neurocytomas do not have processes and the nuclei are more round.

Differential Diagnosis: Choroid Plexus Papilloma

Some ependymomas are papillary, and since both ependymomas and papillomas occur in ventricles, they enter each other's differential diagnosis at times. The papillary structures are different, with a fibrovascular core in choroid plexus tumors (Fig. 4C.15) and a glial center in ependymomas, but this may not be apparent on frozen sections.

Cautions

- All ependymomas are not intraventricular.
- Ependymal "true" rosettes occur in only a small subset of ependymomas.
- Ependymomas cause drop metastases requiring CSF analysis.

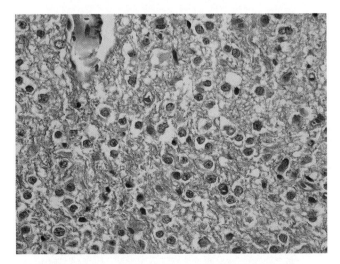

Fig. 4C.14 Histology – neurocytoma – small nuclei with small nucleoli and cleared cytoplasm

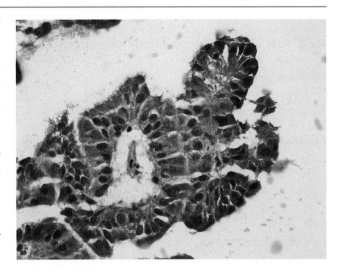

Fig. 4C.15 Histology – choroid plexus papilloma – the fibrovascular core is not showing up well on the frozen sections, the nuclei are larger than ependymal nuclei, tend toward rounder, and have fairly prominent nucleoli

Bibliography

Ependymoma

1. Qian X, Goumnerova LC, De Girolami U, Cibas ES. Cerebrospinal fluid cytology in patients with ependymoma: a bi-institutional retrospective study. Cancer 2008;114(5):307–14.
2. Kim NR, Chung DH, Lee SK, Ha SY. Intramedullary clear cell ependymoma in the thoracic spinal cord: a case with its crush smear and ultrastructural findings. J Korean Med Sci. 2007 Suppl:S149–53.
3. Raisanen J, Burns DK, White CL. Cytology of subependymoma. Acta Cytol. 2003;47(3):518–20.
4. Pai RR, Kini H, Rao VS, Naik R. Choroid plexus papilloma diagnosed by crush cytology. Diagn Cytopathol. 2001;25(3): 165–7.
5. Inayama Y, Nishio Y, Ishii M, Mita K, Motono N, Kawano N, Nakatani Y, Kanno H, Hara M. Crush and imprint cytology of subependymoma: a case report. Acta Cytol. 2001;45(4): 636–40.
6. Otani M, Fujita K, Yokoyama A, Shimizu T, Serizawa H, Kudo M, Ebihara Y. Imprint cytologic features of intracytoplasmic lumina in ependymoma. A report of two cases. Acta Cytol. 2001;45(3): 430–4.
7. Dvoracek MA, Kirby PA. Intraoperative diagnosis of tanycytic ependymoma: pitfalls and differential diagnosis. Diagn Cytopathol. 2001;24(4):289–92.
8. Kumar PV. Nuclear grooves in ependymoma. Cytologic study of 21 cases. Acta Cytol. 1997;41(6):1726–31.
9. Ng HK. Cytologic features of ependymomas in smear preparations. Acta Cytol. 1994;38(3):331–4.

Case 4D
A 60-Year-Old Male with Headache and Ataxia

Cynthia T. Welsh

Clinical History

- 60-year-old male
- Headache and ataxia
- No relevant past medical history
- Exam:
    - Balance problems

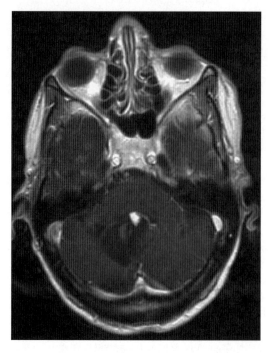

Fig. 4D.2 Axial MRI T1 postcontrast – focal enhancement midline and superior cyst wall; ventricle shifted to left

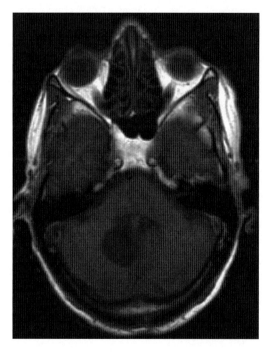

Fig. 4D.1 Axial MRI T1 precontrast – cystic cerebellar tumor just lateral to midline in right hemisphere

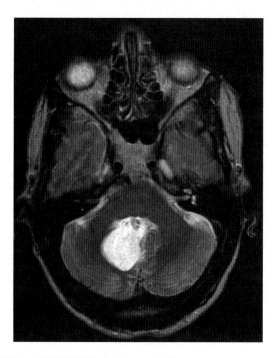

Fig. 4D.3 Axial MRI T2 – bright cyst fluid

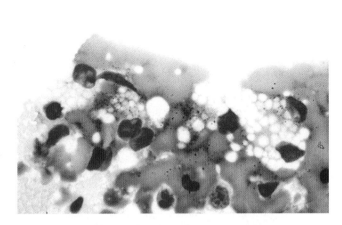

Fig. 4D.4 Smear (H&E stain high magnification) – RBCs and cells with multiple cytoplasmic vacuoles

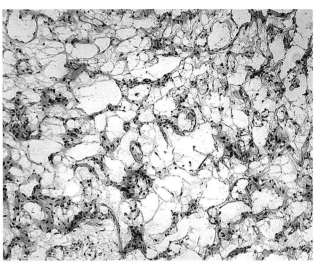

Fig. 4D.6 Frozen section (H&E stain low magnification) – cysts versus freeze artifact

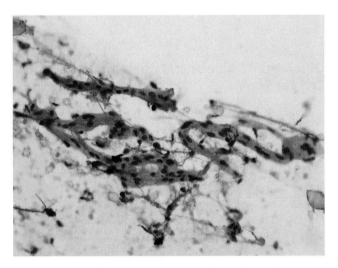

Fig. 4D.5 Smear (H&E stain high magnification) – numerous vessels of various sizes

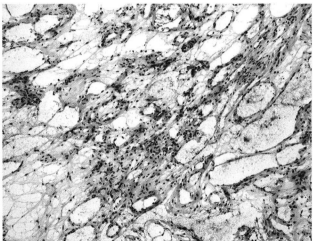

Fig. 4D.7 Frozen section (H&E stain high magnification) – somewhat hyalinized looking vessels and small round nuclei

What Is Your Diagnosis?

Figure Discussion

Scans
Axial sequences show a lesion in the right hemisphere of the cerebellum, which has solid areas that enhance after contrast and has a cyst that is bright on T2. The "cyst with mural nodule" differential (PXA, PA, hemangioblastoma, and ganglioglioma) comes into play (Figs. 4D.1–4D.3).

Pathology
Cysts with mural nodules in the cerebellum are most often pilocytic in children and hemangioblastomas in adults. The histology on frozen section is obscured by the frozen (ice crystal) artifact making everything cystic appearing. The stromal cells on either the frozen or the cytologic preparation suggest hemangioblastoma (Figs. 4D.4–4D.7).

Diagnosis: Hemangioblastoma

Hemangioblastomas are most often cerebellar and sporadic, but may be part of the von Hippel–Lindau (VHL) syndrome (where they can be multiple and extra-cerebellar). The sporadic tumors are seen in adults, but the syndrome-associated tumors may be seen at younger ages. Knowing the history can be very important, and finding that the tumor has associated macrocyst(s) (Table 4D.1) on the scans is also helpful. The patient may have an elevated hematocrit because the tumor produces erythropoietin. Patients with VHL syndrome have a plethora of systemic lesions, with renal cell carcinoma (RCC) among the possibilities, and metastatic RCC is in the differential for vascular tumors with clearing of tumor cell cytoplasm. The first indication grossly that the tumor may be a hemangioblastoma is often the "charred" nature of the specimen. They bleed extensively and cautery is usually used with abandon by the neurosurgeon. The specimen will not squash or smear well. Many vessels of varying calibers will be present. The stromal cells characteristic of the tumor have multiple vacuoles in their cytoplasm filled with lipid. You may want to consider at frozen section cutting extra sections for lipid stains such as Oil Red O stains just in case you need them for more definitive diagnosis later (because of course this will be impossible on the tissue after processing). Scattered large hyperchromatic irregular nuclei are usual in hemangioblastomas, as in many low grade/benign tumors (Table 4D.2). Many of the nuclei will have the cytoplasm stripped from them on smears. The adjacent cerebellum will demonstrate piloid gliosis which will include Rosenthal fiber formation, sometimes of astounding proportions. If the neurosurgeon sends only the reactive cerebellum to you and not the actual tumor, you may think you are dealing with a pilocytic astrocytoma.

Table 4D.1 Cyst with mural nodule

Pilocytic astrocytoma
Hemangioblastoma
Ganglion cell tumors
Pleomorphic xanthoastrocytoma

Table 4D.2 Scattered large irregular hyperchromatic nuclei

Pilocytic astrocytoma
Hemangioblastoma
Meningioma
Schwannoma

Differential Diagnosis: Normal Cerebellum

Normal cerebellum (Fig. 4D.8) doesn't really have any cells that mimic the stromal cell well, but frozen artifact can make virtually any tissue appear to have cleared cells and possible vascular spaces.

Differential Diagnosis: Metastatic Clear Cell Carcinoma

Even in a patient without the history of VHL, RCC is in the differential diagnosis. RCC has a tendency to gravitate to the posterior fossa dura and/or cerebellum when it metastasizes to the CNS. It also is a very vascular tumor and bleeds a lot at surgery. RCC typically has nests outlined by capillary size vessels, and when this distinctive capillary septated pattern is present it favors RCC, but it may be difficult to see on frozen sections (Fig. 4D.9). Although the cells of both tumors have cytoplasmic clearing, the pattern is often different. Hemangioblastoma cells are characterized by multiple bubbles, whereas RCC when "clear cell" has actually cleared out cytoplasm.

Differential Diagnosis: Meningioma

Meningiomas are not uncommon in the posterior fossa and are very vascular, hence the pre-operative embolization to which most of them are subjected. Frozen sections can obscure the features of either tumor, and the specific cell characteristics may be difficult to appreciate (Fig. 4D.10). Neither tumor will squash well. The vessels in meningioma tend to be more often round and hyalinized than those in hemangioblastomas. Meningiomas often have one of a variety of cell types with clear or vacuolated cytoplasm, such as xanthomatous appearing macrophages, but these are usually

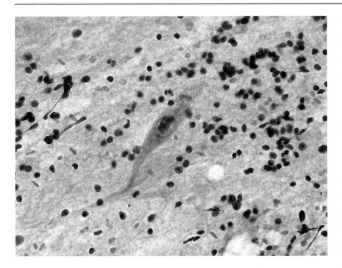

Fig. 4D.8   Smear – normal cerebellum – small internal granular neuronal cells embedded in a neuropil background and a larger Purkinje cell

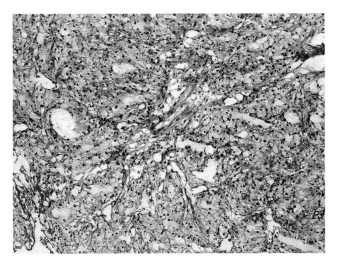

Fig. 4D.9   Histology – metastatic renal cell carcinoma – frozen section artifact obscures the nested architecture and fine capillaries

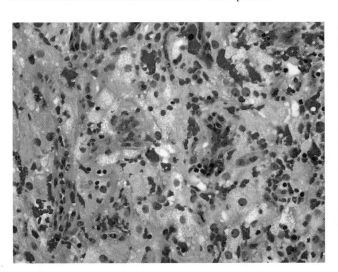

Fig. 4D.10   Histology – meningioma – xanthomatous change and hypervascularity

focal. If none of the meningothelial characteristics (psammoma bodies, pseudoinclusions, etc.) are present, then deferring the diagnosis may be necessary. Both tumors are usually well circumscribed and the surgeon will remove whatever is possible to remove without damage.

Differential Diagnosis: Pilocytic Astrocytoma

While generally a "cyst with mural nodule" in the cerebellum of a child is going to be a pilocytic astrocytoma, in a child with VHL a hemangioblastoma becomes a very viable possibility. Pilocytic tumors do not bleed at surgery the same way, so will not be as cauterized. They can be very vascular under the microscope, however, to the point sometimes of simulating vascular malformations. The microcystic nature of the looser areas in pilocytic astrocytomas (Fig. 4D.11) may resemble the stromal cells of hemangioblastoma. Cerebellar pilocytic astrocytomas have oligodendroglial-like cells which enter the differential for cleared cell tumors also. If the neurosurgeon sends only the reactive cerebellum around a hemangioblastoma to you, you may think you are dealing with a pilocytic astrocytoma. Fortunately, piloid gliosis is generally far less cellular and demonstrates far more Rosenthal fibers than the actual pilocytic astrocytoma usually does.

Differential Diagnosis: Vascular Malformation

Generally, cerebellar vascular malformations (Fig. 4D.12), and the piloid type of gliosis that you might see around them in this location, would more commonly be in the differential with pilocytic astrocytomas. On occasion they might be confused with hemangioblastoma, but will lack the stromal cells.

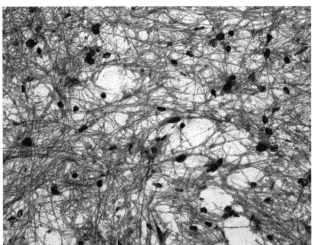

Fig. 4D.11   Histology – pilocytic astrocytoma – prominent network of processes giving the impression of possibly encircling vacuolated cells

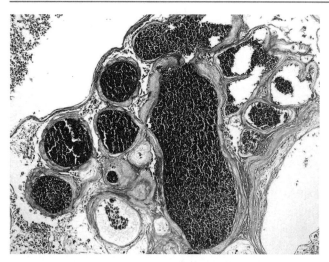

Fig. 4D.12 Histology – angioma – back to back blood vessels without any bubbly stromal cells

Cautions

Cerebellum adjacent to hemangioblastomas is cellular, gliotic, and acquires Rosenthal fibers.

Bibliography

Hemangioblastoma

1. Xiong J, Chu SG, Wang Y, Zhu JJ, Li C, Mao Y. Metastasis of renal cell carcinoma to a haemangioblastoma of the medulla oblongata in von Hippel-Lindau syndrome. J Clin Neurosci. 2010;17(9):1213–5.
2. Lallu S, Naran S, Palmer D, Bethwaite P. Cyst fluid cytology of cerebellar hemangioblastoma: a case report. Diagn Cytopathol. 2008; 36(5):341–3.
3. Ortega L, Jiménez-Heffernan JA, Perna C. Squash cytology of cerebellar haemangioblastoma. Cytopathology 2002;13(3):184–5.
4. Commins DL, Hinton DR. Cytologic features of hemangioblastoma: comparison with meningioma, anaplastic astrocytoma and renal cell carcinoma. Acta Cytol. 1998;42(5):1104–10.
5. Yamamoto T, Wakui K, Kobayashi M. Hemangioblastoma in the cerebellar vermis: a case report. Acta Cytol. 1996;40(2):346–50.
6. Silverman JF, Dabbs DJ, Leonard JR 3rd, Harris LS. Fine needle aspiration cytology of hemangioblastoma of the spinal cord. Report of a case with immunocytochemical and ultrastructural studies. Acta Cytol. 1986;30(3):303–8.

Case 4E
A 30-Year-Old Female with Headaches and Visual Changes

M. Timothy Smith

Clinical History

- 30-year-old female
- 2 weeks progressive headache, double vision, nausea, vomiting
- Exam:
  - Slight dysmetria
  - Depressed reflexes

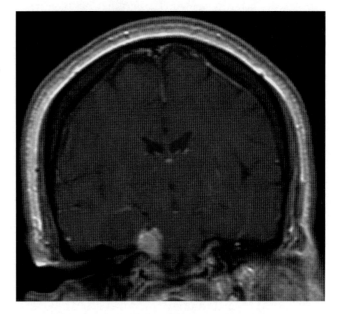

Fig. 4E.2 Coronal T1 MRI postcontrast – the tumor enhance homogeneously and there is a suggestion of a dural tail

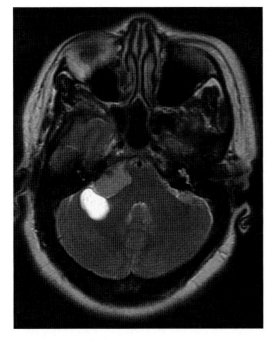

Fig. 4E.1 Axial T2 MRI – right cerebellopontine angle (CPA) tumor brighter than brain, adjacent cyst fluid very bright

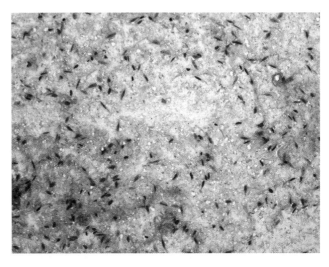

Fig. 4E.3 Smear (H&E stain high magnification) – the lesion smears well and demonstrates individual cells with elongate nuclei in a vacuolated background

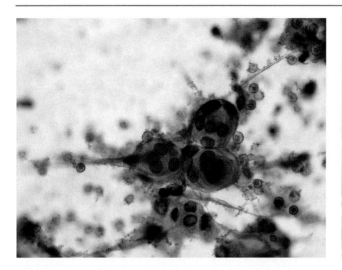

Fig. 4E.4 Smear (H&E stain high magnification) – tight whirls of cells with central mineralization

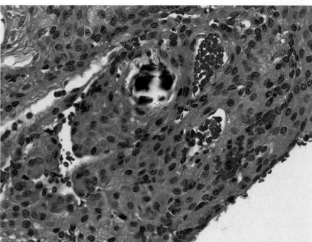

Fig. 4E.6 Frozen section (H&E stain high magnification) – calcification and small round to oval nuclei

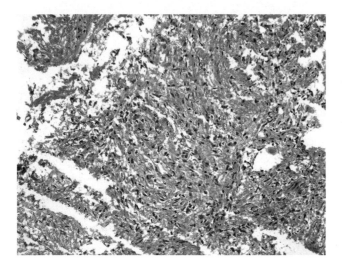

Fig. 4E.5 Frozen section (H&E stain low magnification) – the elongate nuclei are seen in the frozen section along with pink globular cytoplasm similar to gemistocytes

What Is Your Diagnosis?

Figure Discussion

Scans

The cyst might suggest schwannoma over meningioma but there is no internal auditory canal component, and though not specific, the dural tail supports a meningioma (Figs. 4E.1–4E.2).

Pathology

One of the smears and one of the frozen sections show very nonspecific bland spindle cells, the others show the cellular whirls of a meningioma, oval nuclei, and psammoma bodies. The hyalinized vessels typical of meningioma are not seen in these portions of the specimen (Figs. 4E.3–4E.6).

Diagnosis: Meningioma

The most common supratentorial extra-axial tumor in an adult is meningioma, unless there is a history of malignant systemic tumor in which case metastatic disease rises considerably in the differential. The differential diagnosis in the cerebellopontine angle (CPA) is dominated by schwannomas, but there are other possibilities (especially meningioma). The difference on scans is partly highlighted by involvement of the internal auditory canal (more likely schwannoma) versus demonstration of a dural tail (more likely meningioma). The pattern of enhancement and presence of a cystic component also can help. Both meningiomas and schwannomas can be spindle cell lesions without distinguishing characteristics (as seen in the figures in this case), especially on frozen sections. Neither one will typically smear well, but around the edges of the smear you may be able to see structures not seen on the frozen that help to identify a meningeal quality to the lesion. On the other hand, this may be a good opportunity to stop the cytologic preparation when the tissue won't squash, and instead to do multiple touch preparations. These will generally show you better morphology of small groups than you will be able to see if you had continued to try to smear the tissue. Whirls of cells and psammoma bodies are not exclusive to meningiomas, as normal arachnoid/leptomeninges form these also. Vessels are hyalinized and tend to be round, and not at all slit-like. If no specific patterns are seen, the intraoperative diagnosis may be only "spindle cell lesion" or possibly "spindle cell neoplasm" and may or may not include a probable grade. This generally will not affect the planned surgery. Some variants of meningioma resemble other tumors such as chordoid and rhabdoid variants which obviously are similar to chordoma (Fig. 4E.7) and rhabdoid (Fig. 4E.8) tumors respectively, and bring those tumors into the differential. Secretory meningiomas (Fig. 4E.9) can be confused with metastatic carcinomas such as thyroid (Fig. 4E.10). Pituitary adenomas can have psammoma bodies (Fig. 4E.11) like meningiomas.

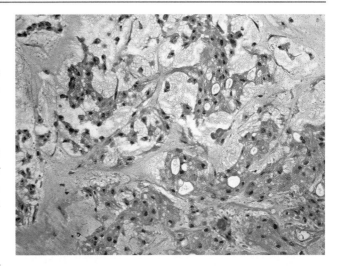

Fig. 4E.7 Histology – chordoma – cords of eosinophilic cells in a myxoid background

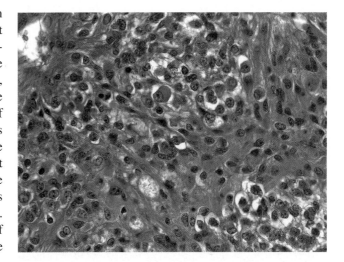

Fig. 4E.8 Histology – rhabdoid tumor – dense eosinophilic cytoplasmic bodies and pleomorphic eccentric nuclei

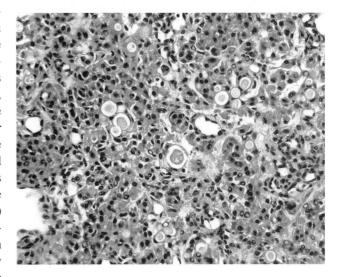

Fig. 4E.9 Histology – secretory meningioma – pseudopsammoma bodies and numerous intranuclear cytoplasmic pseudoinclusions

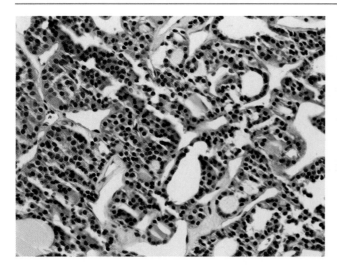

Fig. 4E.10 Histology – thyroid metastasis – follicles with colloid and fairly bland cells. No intranuclear inclusions are seen in this particular frozen section

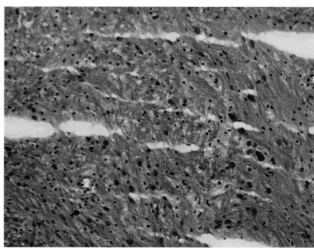

Fig. 4E.12 Histology – schwannoma – nondescript, almost glial appearing tissue without obvious schwannian structures, and occasional large irregular, hyperchromatic nuclei

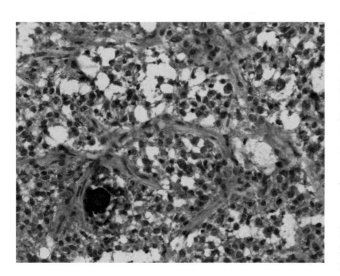

Fig. 4E.11 Histology – pituitary adenoma – nesting, vacuolation of cells, and a psammoma body

Differential Diagnosis: Schwannoma

Both meningiomas and schwannomas (Fig. 4E.12) can be spindle cell lesions without distinguishing characteristics, especially on frozen sections. Either can be very similar to glial tissue (except usually not squashing/smearing well). Both tumors contain hyalinized blood vessels and may demonstrate hemosiderin-laden macrophages, degenerative cystic areas, a biphasic appearance, and mast cell infiltration, but all of the latter favor schwannoma. Scattered enlarged, irregular, hyperchromatic nuclei are another

degenerative feature that these two tumors have in common. If Verocay bodies are present, then the lesion is most likely a schwannoma. These are not seen in meningiomas, but are present in other soft tissue tumors (which seldom develop within the CNS). As mentioned above, the cytologic preparations may sometimes be of more use than the frozen sections in differentiating between the schwannomas and meningiomas.

Differential Diagnosis: Hemangiopericytoma

Hemangiopericytomas are usually presented to you by the neurosurgeon as a meningioma, but the neuroradiologist may have some idea that hemangiopericytoma is in the differential because of the more prominent vascular channels on scans. The frozen will show a spindle cell tumor (Fig. 4E.13) which will typically be more cellular than usual for a meningioma. The vessels will be slit-like (staghorn) rather than hyalinized, which will be your first clue at low power that you are looking at something different than a meningioma. Either the frozen or the cytologic preparations (Fig. 4E.14) can show you how much more mitotically active the hemangiopericytoma often is than the usual meningioma. The nuclei are generally more round with denser chromatin on smears than meningiomas. Less cytoplasm is usually seen on smears of hemangiopericytomas. In sections, the nuclei tend to be more vesicular and irregular in appearance. It may be helpful to the neurosurgeon to know intraoperatively that hemangiopericytoma is in the differential, as it may affect the extent of resection.

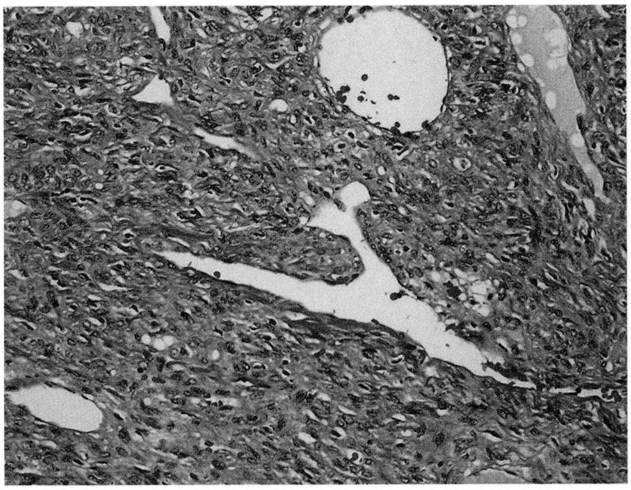

Fig. 4E.13 Histology – hemangiopericytoma – slit-like vasculature, vesicular overlapping nuclei, multiple mitoses, and small nucleoli

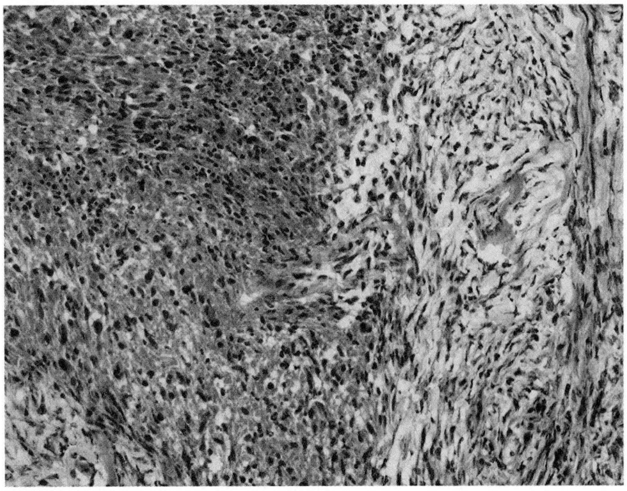

Fig. 4E.15 Histology – gliosarcoma – almost a biphasic appearance (more and less dense areas) of spindle cells

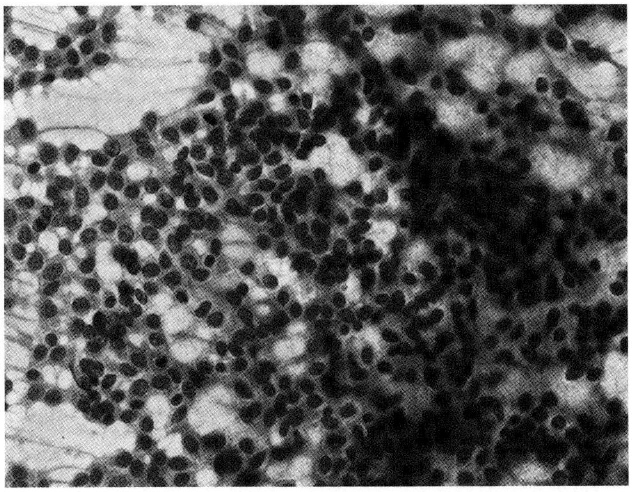

Fig. 4E.14 Smear – hemangiopericytoma – borders around somewhat polygonal appearing cells, which seem to have some attachments between cells. Salt and pepper chromatin, tiny nucleoli, fairly monotonous but several mitotic figures are present

Differential Diagnosis: Gliosarcoma

Superficial high-grade glial neoplasms involving leptomeninges and having a spindle cell component (Fig. 4E.15) can be difficult to separate from meningiomas invading brain. Both of the spindle cell lesions typical to the CPA (schwannoma and meningioma) may resemble glial tissue on frozen sections. Often the lack of smearing on the cytology will make it obvious that you aren't actually dealing with the usual glial tissue, but "sarcomatous" transformation doesn't smear well either. Neoplastic astrocytes will be your best indication that the process is actually glial.

Cautions

- Psammoma bodies can be seen in normal or reactive (hyperplastic) leptomeninges and in subtypes of pituitary adenoma (know your location!).
- Meningiomas occur in spots where other tumors are more common, such as the CPA or inside ventricles.

Bibliography

Meningioma

1. Xiao GQ, Burstein DE. Cytologic findings of rhabdoid meningioma in cerebrospinal fluid. Acta Cytol. 2008;52(1):118–9.
2. Nicolas MM, Kaakaji R, Russell EJ, De Frias DV, Nayar R. Extradural spinal meningioma as a source of plasmacytoid cells. A case report. Acta Cytol. 2007;51(1):68–72.
3. Inagawa H, Ishizawa K, Shimada S, Shimada T, Nishikawa R, Matsutani M, Hirose T. Cytologic features of chordoid meningioma. A case report. Acta Cytol. 2004;48(3):397–401.
4. Salinero E, Beltran L, Costa JR. Intraoperative cytologic diagnosis of chordoid meningioma. A case report. Acta Cytol. 2004;48(2):259–63.
5. Kirby PA. Rhabdoid meningioma: intraoperative diagnosis using smear preparation. Diagn Cytopathol. 2003;29(5):292–6.
6. Pope LZ, Tatsui CE, Moro MS, Neto AC, Bleggi-Torres LF. Meningioma with extensive noncalcifying collagenous whorls and glial fibrillary acidic protein expression: new variant of meningioma diagnosed by smear preparation. Diagn Cytopathol. 2003;28(5):274–7.
7. Ghosal N, Kapila K, Sharma MC, Verma K. Fine needle aspiration cytology of a meningioma with extracranial extension after irradiation for medulloblastoma. Acta Cytol. 2001;45(6):1092–3.
8. Fukuoka K, Hirokawa M, Kanahara T, Ishii N, Ishii R, Shirabe T. Cytology of microcystic meningioma in crush preparation. Diagn Cytopathol. 2000;23(4):275–8.
9. Hinton DR, Kovacs K, Chandrasoma PT. Cytologic features of secretory meningioma. Acta Cytol. 1999;43(2):121–5.

The Base of Skull (Including Pineal and Sella Turcica Regions) Lesion

5

Case 5A
A 27-Year-Old Female with Visual Disturbance and Headaches

Cynthia T. Welsh

Clinical History

- 27-year-old female
- Visual disturbance
- Headaches
- Exam:
    - Visual field defect

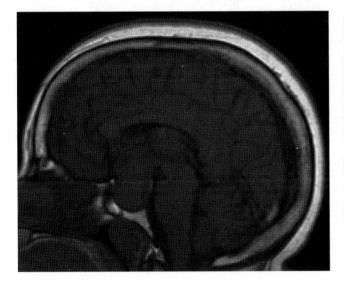

Fig. 5A.1 Sagittal MRI T1 precontrast – intrasellar and suprasellar mass

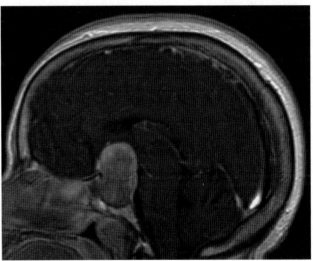

Fig. 5A.2 Sagittal MRI T1 postcontrast – enhancing intrasellar and suprasellar mass

C.T. Welsh (✉)
Department of Pathology and Laboratory Medicine,
Medical University of South Carolina, Charleston, SC 29425, USA
e-mail: welshct@musc.edu

C.T. Welsh (ed.), *Intra-Operative Neuropathology for the Non-Neuropathologist: A Case-Based Approach*,
DOI 10.1007/978-1-4419-1167-4_5, © Springer Science+Business Media, LLC 2012

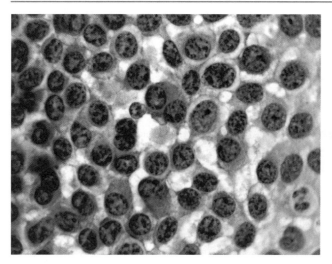

Fig. 5A.3 Touch preparation (H&E stain high magnification) – eccentric nuclei with chromatin clumping and occasional red nucleoli; occasional binucleate cells

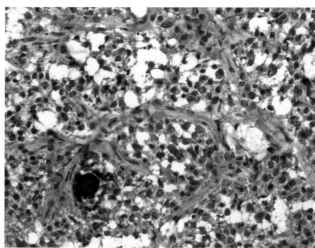

Fig. 5A.5 Frozen section (H&E stain high magnification) – occasional small nest of cells, but otherwise sheets, occasional laminated microcalcification; some cells display the eccentric nucleus which was seen much better on cytology

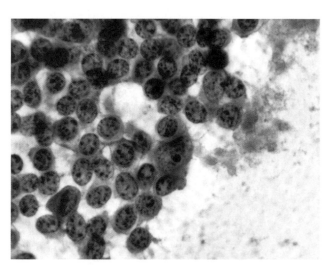

Fig. 5A.4 Touch preparation (H&E stain high magnification) – occasional larger cells are seen

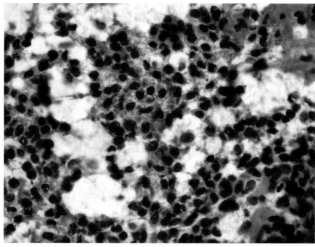

Fig. 5A.6 Frozen section (H&E stain high magnification) – sheets of cells, some variation in nuclear size (less in shape)

What Is Your Diagnosis?

Figure Discussion

Scans
This tumor sits in the sella which is enlarged and is also suprasellar. It fairly homogeneously enhances (Figs. 5A.1–5A.2).

Pathology
The touch preparations show monotonous round nuclei with small nucleoli, and eccentric eosinophilic cytoplasm. Occasional cells are binucleate. The chromatin is coarsely clumped. One of the tissue sections demonstrates nesting and a laminated microcalcification like a meningeal psammoma body. While these cells are plasmacytoid, they are also very bland consistent with an adenoma (Figs. 5A.3–5A.6).

Diagnosis: Pituitary Adenoma

Pituitary tumors are almost all benign adenomas. Many of these are treated medically first, and only surgically resected when medical therapy fails. Fortunately, the medical therapy does not usually alter the pathology sufficiently to make diagnosis difficult. What does make it challenging sometimes is the tiny size of the specimen and the crush artifact. Frozen section diagnosis rests on finding sheets of cells instead of normal anterior pituitary nests. Small sample size may make pattern recognition difficult. Touch preparations can obviate this problem entirely. Touch preparations do not take anything appreciable away from the histologic sample. They actually give you more information than a squash/smear does. The normal reticulin network of the anterior pituitary holds cells tightly into the nested framework. An adenoma does not have this reticulin framework, so numerous cells stick to the slide, compared to normal anterior pituitary which leaves behind few cells on a touch prep. Just remember to do multiple touches on the slide so the RBCs come off the surface, then the tumor cells can show you a good cell button. Most pituitary adenomas have monotonous small cells with eccentric nuclei, occasional binucleate cells, rare mitoses, and little pleomorphism. Nucleoli are small and infrequent. Adenomas have many different morphologies (partly depending on which hormone they make) and may demonstrate perivascular pseudorosettes, papillary structure, dense round "fibrous" bodies in cytoplasm, psammoma body-like calcifications, cords of cells, clear cells, or make amyloid.

Differential Diagnosis: Normal Anterior Pituitary

The material sent from neurosurgeons performing a pituitary surgery via the sphenoid sinus often includes some anterior pituitary and possible posterior pituitary as well. The normal nested structure of a mixture of cell types in the anterior pitu-

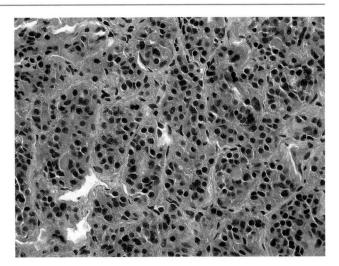

Fig. 5A.7 Histology – normal anterior pituitary – normal nesting somewhat obscured by artifact. Most of the cells have no obvious granules; a few are eosinophilic

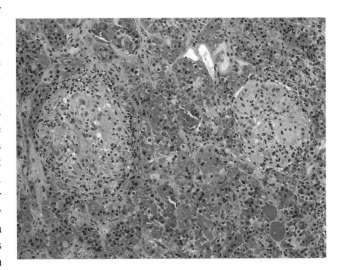

Fig. 5A.8 Histology – sarcoid in anterior pituitary – "naked" granulomas in eosinophilic cells

itary (Fig. 5A.7) on frozen section can be much harder to recognize because of things such as the degranulation of normal cells during freezing (making them deceptively homogeneous looking), and masking of normal nesting by the crushing/cautery incident to surgery. Normal anterior pituitary has many cyst-like structures such as Rathkes cleft cysts and follicle or gland-like formation. Pituitary involved by inflammatory processes such as sarcoid (Fig. 5A.8) may resemble a neoplasm on scans and frozen sections.

Differential Diagnosis: Meningioma

Psammoma body-like calcifications and pseudoinclusions not only occur in meningiomas but also in certain subtypes of pituitary adenomas. Meningiomas are more common

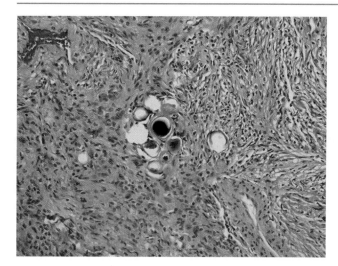

Fig. 5A.9 Histology – meningioma – whirls of oval cells with intra-nuclear cytoplasmic pseudoinclusions and a psammoma body

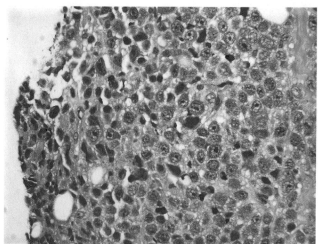

Fig. 5A.10 Histology – myeloma – very immature plasma cells with large vesicular nuclei and prominent nucleoli, no plasmacytoid characteristics to the chromatin, and rarely enough cytoplasm to be considered eccentric

over the convexities, but not uncommon at the skull base. Meningiomas do not give you a nice cell button on touch preparations like pituitary adenomas, but some small cell groups usually adhere to the slide. The whirls of meningothelial cells (Fig. 5A.9), if present, help to define the meningioma.

Differential Diagnosis: Plasma Cell Dyscrasia

Pituitary adenomas can have a decidedly plasmacytoid morphology which can be disconcerting to the unaware, especially considering the proximity of the skull base which is a potential source for plasma cell lesions. Plasma cells and pituitary cells can both show eccentric nuclei, mitoses, and scattered binucleate cells. A suggestion of a Hoff is often seen in pituitary adenoma cells. The clock face chromatin pattern of normal/reactive plasma cells may not be very apparent, less so as the cells become more immature. Plasma cell dyscrasias tend to show more binucleate cells, more mitoses, and real Hoffs (Fig. 5A.10) compared to pituitary adenomas.

Differential Diagnosis: Germ Cell Tumors

Small or large monotonous cells in the sella or suprasellar region in a child are more likely to be something other than a pituitary adenoma. Sella is one of the midline predilections of germ cell tumors (Fig. 5A.11). The morphology is of course going to depend on the subtypes of germ cell tumor, any of which may be present.

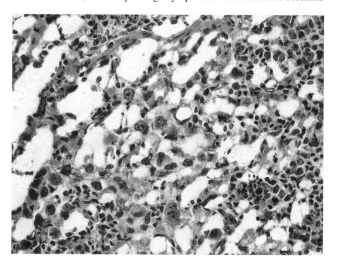

Fig. 5A.11 Histology – germinoma – background lymphocytes and scattered large cells with large nuclei, prominent nucleoli, and variable cytoplasm

Differential Diagnosis:– Metastatic Tumor

Renal cell carcinoma (RCC) metastases (Fig. 5A.12) can be nested like pituitary. Crush artifact in a pituitary adenoma can mimic metastatic small cell carcinoma. Thyroid tumor metastases (Fig. 5A.13) can be monotonous and fairly bland unlike a lot of metastatic tumors which are more obviously malignant. A history of any head/neck tumor makes it a very clear contender in the differential diagnosis.

Differential Diagnosis: Pituicytoma

Pituicytomas tend more toward spindle cells (Fig. 5A.14). They are monotonous, bland bipolar cells with oval nuclei. They may appear fascicular.

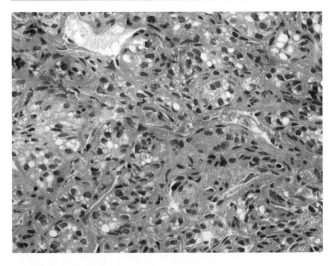

Fig. 5A.12 Histology – metastatic renal cell carcinoma – nests of cells with vacuolated cytoplasm

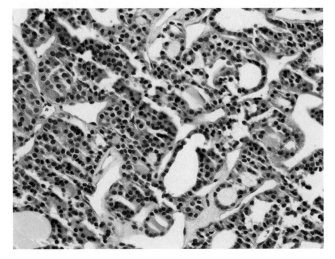

Fig. 5A.13 Histology – metastatic thyroid carcinoma – small round to oval, monotonous nuclei with no pleomorphism or mitoses – follicular structure with colloid apparent in some of the spaces

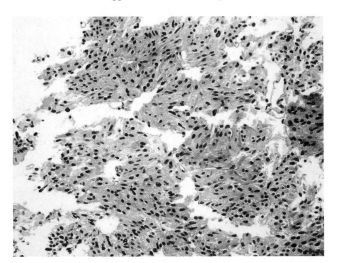

Fig. 5A.14 Histology – pituicytoma – spindle cells with oval nuclei, no atypia, and no mitoses

Cautions

- All laminated microcalcifications are not meningeal psammoma bodies.
- Pituitary adenoma cells can have intranuclear pseudoinclusions.
- Many pituitary adenoma cells are binucleate and have eccentric nuclei similar to plasma cells.
- Nuclear atypia does not make a pituitary tumor carcinoma.
- Freezing anterior pituitary degranulates the cells making them appear monotonous.

Bibliography

Pituitary Adenoma

1. Policarpio-Nicolas ML, Le BH, Mandell JW, Lopes MB. Granular cell tumor of the neurohypophysis: report of a case with intraoperative cytologic diagnosis. Diagn Cytopathol. 2008;36(1): 58–63.
2. Takei H, Buckleair L, Goodman JC, Powell SZ. Intraoperative cytologic diagnosis of symptomatic carcinoma (pulmonary small cell carcinoma) metastatic to the pituitary gland: a case report. Acta Cytol. 2007;51(4):637–41.
3. Ghosal N, Satish R, Menon S, Hegde AS, Santosh V. Pituitary adenoma-neuronal choristoma (PANCH): cytomorphology on smear preparation. Cytopathology. 2006;17(3):149–52.
4. Kobayashi TK, Bamba M, Oka H, Hino A, Fujimoto M, Katsumori T, Moritani S, Kushima R, Kaneko C. Granular cell tumour of the neurohypophysis on cytological squash preparations. Cytopathology. 2006;17(3):153–4.
5. Chen KT. Crush cytology of pituicytoma. Diagn Cytopathol. 2005;33(4):255–7.
6. Inagawa H, Ishizawa K, Mitsuhashi T, Shimizu M, Adachi J, Nishikawa R, Matsutani M, Hirose T. Giant invasive pituitary adenoma extending into the sphenoid sinus and nasopharynx: report of a case with intraoperative cytologic diagnosis. Acta Cytol. 2005; 49(4):452–6.
7. Madhavan M, P JG, Abdullah Jafri J, Idris Z. Intraventricular squamous papillary craniopharyngioma: report of a case with intraoperative imprint cytology. Acta Cytol. 2005;49(4):431–4.
8. Tanboon J, Chaipipat M, Wattanasirmkit V, Wongtabtim W, Shuangshoti S, Bunyaratavej K. Squash cytology of Rosai-Dorfman disease in the sellar region. Acta Cytol. 2003;47(6):1143–4.
9. Smith AR, Elsheikh TM, Silverman JF. Intraoperative cytologic diagnosis of suprasellar and sellar cystic lesions. Diagn Cytopathol. 1999;20(3):137–47.

Case 5B
A 56-Year-Old Female with Headache, Dizziness, Double Vision

Cynthia T. Welsh

Clinical History

- 56-year-old female
- Headaches, nausea/vomiting, dizziness, double vision
- Exam:
  - Sixth nerve palsy

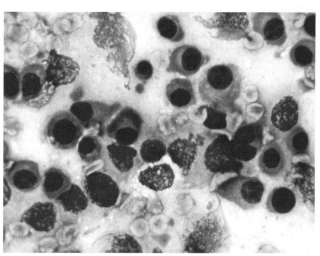

Fig. 5B.3 Touch preparation (DQ stain high magnification) – a cell population which has smudgy nuclei, and one with eccentric cytoplasm and perinuclear cytoplasmic clearing

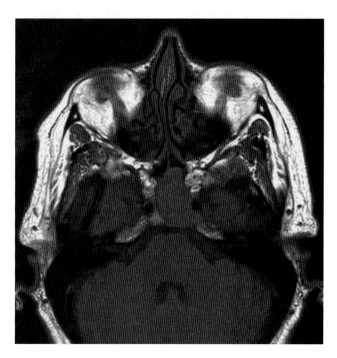

Fig. 5B.1 Axial T1 MRI – midline mass with left cavernous sinus invasion (wrapped around carotid)

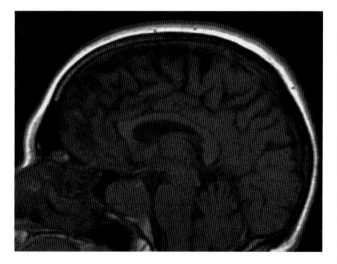

Fig. 5B.2 Sagittal midline T1 MRI – mass in clivus, sella, and suprasellar space

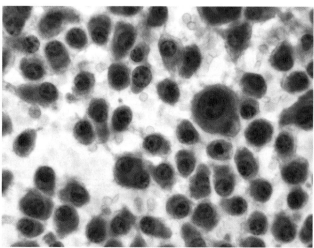

Fig. 5B.4 Touch preparation (H&E stain high magnification) – eccentric nuclei with clumped chromatin, nuclear membrane accentuation, and occasional binucleate cells

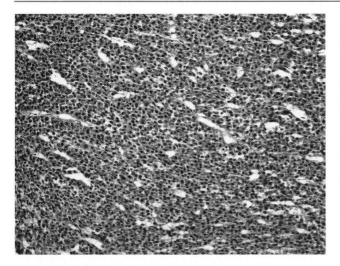

Fig. 5B.5 Frozen section (H&E stain low magnification) – sheets of cells

Fig. 5B.6   Frozen section (H&E stain high magnification) – eccentric nuclei, perinuclear cytoplasmic clearing

What Is Your Diagnosis?

Figure Discussion

Scans
There is a midline clivus mass with left cavernous sinus and sella invasion and obvious bone destruction (Figs. 5B.1–5B.2).

Pathology
Eccentric nuclei with clumped chromatin, nuclear membrane accentuation, and occasional binucleate cells on the H&E stained smear. The perinuclear golgi clearings, "Hoffs," show best on the Diff Quik stained smear. Sheets of cells are seen on the tissue sections. These cells are mature enough to obviously be plasma cells, and there are increased numbers (Figs. 5B.3–5B.6).

Diagnosis: Plasmacytoma

The sella is one of the places that neurosurgeons tend to tell you where they are. Just because the paperwork you have says sella though doesn't mean that the lesion isn't actually "sellar region," which can mean a lot of things. If it is actually the clivus/skull base involved, then the differential turns to bone lesions such as plasmacytoma/myeloma, chordoma, metastatic or locally invasive head/neck tumors, or (in childhood) Langerhans cell lesions, instead of sellar/suprasellar tumors such as pituitary adenoma, craniopharyngioma, and germ cell tumors. Plasmacytomas can occur as solitary lytic bone lesions (skull or vertebra), or as part of multiple myeloma. They may also be dural based. The patients are usually older adults. The differential frequently involves a chronic inflammatory (lymphoplasmacytoid) reactive infiltrate. The characteristic chromatin "clockface" and eccentric cytoplasm with perinuclear "Hoffs" make the diagnosis. Plasma cells lesions generally have more mitoses and binucleate cells than pituitary tumors. The neoplastic plasma cells may be so immature as to be difficult to recognize as plasma cells; knowing the radiologic characteristics may be what leads you to think of the possibility.

Differential Diagnosis: Pituitary Adenoma

Frequently, pituitary adenoma cells are binucleate like plasma cells, but there are usually fewer binucleate cells. Multinucleate cells, which are not uncommon in plasma cell dyscrasias, are rare in pituitary. Adenomas may have mitoses, but fewer than you expect in a plasma cell lesion. Often the nucleus is eccentric as in plasma cells, but the chromatin pattern is different (Fig. 5B.7). Although neoplastic plasma cells lose the clockface of normal/reactive plasma cells, the chromatin remains more clumped than seen in pituitary nuclei. There is frequently

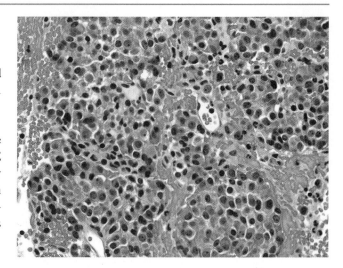

Fig. 5B.7 Touch preparation – pituitary adenoma – single cells with eccentric eosinophilic cytoplasm, fairly large round nuclei, prominent nucleoli, and occasional binucleate cells

the suggestion of a "Hoff" in adenomas that have eccentric nuclei, but it will be better defined (real) in the plasma cells.

Differential Diagnosis: Meningioma

Meningiomas are not uncommon along the skull base and their nuclei can be eccentric like plasma cells. Most meningiomas squash and smear poorly, but the occasional one will smear well and can be confused with something nonmeningeal. One hopes to see psammoma bodies and/or one of the patterns typical for meningioma (Fig. 5B.8), and the typical meningothelial nuclei (round to oval with pseudoinclusions).

Differential Diagnosis: Metastases

Metastases and direct invasion of the skull base or basal dura happens in a number of tumors. A plasmacytoid appearance (especially in frozen sections) can be mimicked by the basal lamina accumulations in some salivary gland tumors (Fig. 5B.9), many of which like to crawl up into the cranium by way of nerves.

Differential Diagnosis: Germ Cell Tumors

The sella/suprasellar region and pineal area are the common sites for germ cell tumors, and so are in areas at the skullbase near where plasma cell lesions occur. The most common germ cell tumors in the differential with plasma cell lesions would be the ones which tend to demonstrate large single cells such as germinomas (Fig. 5B.10) and embryonal carcinomas, but these groups of tumors occur in different age groups.

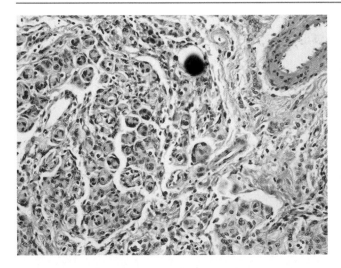

Fig. 5B.8 Histology – meningioma – multiple whirls of cells, intra-nuclear cytoplasmic pseudoinclusions, and one psammoma body

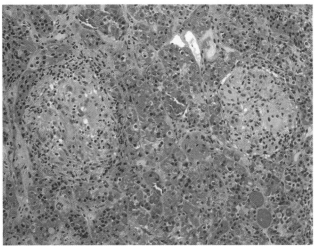

Fig. 5B.11 Histology – sarcoid – "naked" granulomas in anterior pituitary

Differential Diagnosis: Other

Hypophysitis and sarcoid (Fig. 5B.11) tend to disrupt normal pituitary to the point where it becomes difficult to recognize and can look like tumor.

Cautions

- Plasma cells can be increased in chronic inflammatory conditions.
- Plasma cells may be so immature as to be difficult to recognize unless you know there is a lytic bone lesion putting plasmacytoma into the differential.
- Pituitary adenomas and meningiomas can be plasmacytoid.

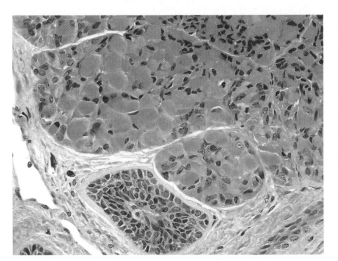

Fig. 5B.9 Histology – salivary gland neoplasm – basal lamina material making nuclei eccentric and mimicking Russell bodies

Bibliography

Plasmacytoma

1. Pitini V, Arrigo C, Alafaci C, Altavilla G. Extramedullary plasmacytoma presented as a non-functional invasive pituitary macroadenoma. J Neurooncol. 2008;88(2):227–9.
2. Licci S, Narciso P. Myelomatous meningitis. Eur J Haematol. 2008;81(4):328.
3. Nicolas MM, Kaakaji R, Russell EJ, De Frias DV, Nayar R. Extradural spinal meningioma as a source of plasmacytoid cells. A case report. Acta Cytol. 2007;51(1):68–72.
4. Khayyata S, Bentley G, Fregene TA, Al-Abbadi M. Retroperitoneal extramedullary anaplastic plasmacytoma masquerading as sarcoma: report of a case with an unusual presentation and imprint smears. Acta Cytol. 2007;51(3):434–6.
5. Nassar DL, Raab SS, Silverman JF, Kennerdell JS, Sturgis CD. Fine-needle aspiration for the diagnosis of orbital hematolymphoid lesions. Diagn Cytopathol. 2000;23(5):314–7.
6. Aboul-Nasr R, Estey EH, Kantarjian HM, Freireich EJ, Andreeff M, Johnson BJ, Albitar M. Comparison of touch imprints with aspirate smears for evaluating bone marrow specimens. Am J Clin Pathol. 1999;111(6):753–8.

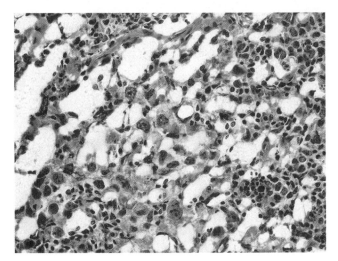

Fig. 5B.10 Histology – germinoma – lymphocytic background with scattered large cells with large mostly round nuclei and prominent nucleoli

Case 5C
A 55-Year-Old Male with Complaints of Swallowing Difficulties

Cynthia T. Welsh

Clinical History

- 55-year-old male
- Complaint of abnormal tongue, swallowing difficulty
- Exam:
  - Right hypoglossal nerve paralysis

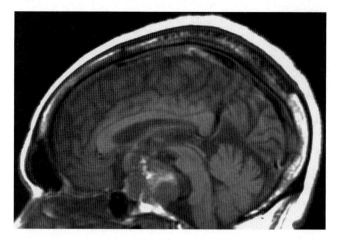

Fig. 5C.2 Sagittal MRI T1 precontrast – midline changes in clivus with pons compression, and mixed density including central hyperdense areas

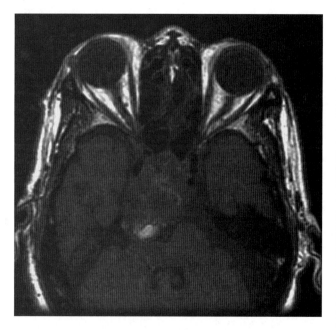

Fig. 5C.1 Axial MRI T1 precontrast – midline changes in clivus (although there is some right sided extension), with mixed density, possibly cystic areas

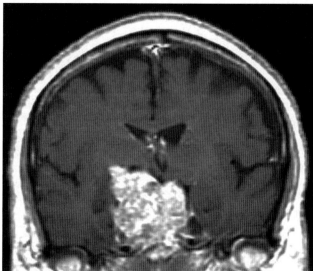

Fig. 5C.3 Coronal MRI T1 postcontrast – heterogeneously enhancing tumor pushing brain upward

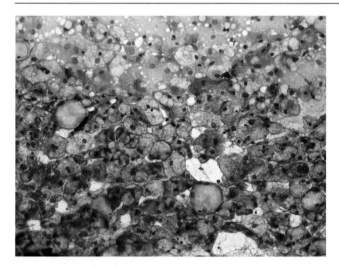

Fig. 5C.4 Smear (H&E stain low magnification) – small nuclei and abundant cytoplasm which ranges from eosinophilic to bubbly (one to multiple vacuoles

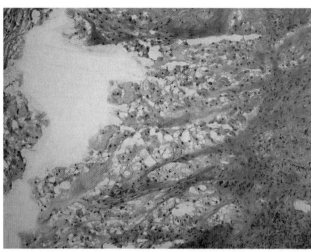

Fig. 5C.6 Frozen section (H&E stain low magnification) – nests of cells with bubbly or eosinophilic cytoplasm and small nuclei; myxoid background, and hemosiderin-laden macrophages

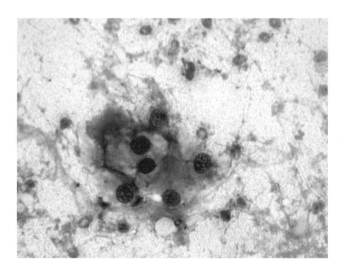

Fig. 5C.5 Smear (DQ stain high magnification) – round nuclei, abundant cytoplasm

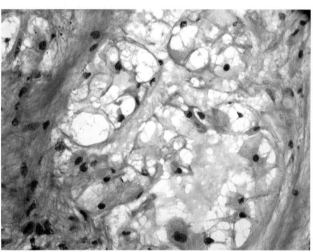

Fig. 5C.7 Frozen section (H&E stain high magnification) – closer view of nests of cells with bubbly or eosinophilic cytoplasm and small nuclei; myxoid background, and hemosiderin-laden macrophages

What Is Your Diagnosis?

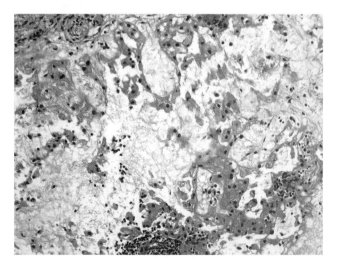

Fig. 5C.8 Frozen section (H&E stain low magnification) – cords of cells with eosinophilic cytoplasm

Figure Discussion

Scans

A midline skullbase bone lesion arising from the clivus with heterogeneous enhancement and probable cystic areas (Figs. 5C.1–5C.3).

Pathology

Cords of eosinophilic cells, cells with multiple vacuoles (physaliferous cells) and a myxoid background. There are lobules of cells on the tissue sections. The combination of location, cell types, and myxoid background is consistent with the diagnosis of chordoma (Figs. 5C.4–5C.8).

Diagnosis: Chordoma

Chordomas tend to occur near both ends of the vertebral column, in clivus or sacrum, and rarely in between. There is a male predominance. Cranial nerve signs, visual symptoms, and pain are common due to location in the skull base lesions; whereas, the sacral lesions cause pain and spinal nerve compression. A "bubbly" appearance can often be seen on scans. CT shows the calcifications and bone destruction best. There is enhancement and they are bright on T2 MRI. The tumors demonstrate both eosinophilic cytoplasm and "bubbly" (physaliferous) cells. Sections show a nested pattern (lobules with septations) and a myxoid (Table 5C.1) or chondroid background. Occasional large hyperchromatic nuclei are common, but necrosis, mitoses, and pleomorphism are unusual. Intraoperatively the tumors with a chondroid background will probably have to be termed "low grade cartilaginous" neoplasms and further differentiation from chondrosarcoma done on permanent sections with possibly immunohistochemistry.

Differential Diagnosis: Chondrosarcoma

Chondrosarcomas are generally lateral, rather than midline like chordoma. The chondroid variant of chordoma in particular looks very similar to chondrosarcoma (Fig. 5C.9). These are different tumors with different prognosis and treatment. In order not to cloud the issue of which tumor it is, it is frequently a reasonable idea to keep the intraoperative diagnosis general rather than specific such as "low-grade myxoid and/or chondroid neoplasm."

Table 5C.1 Myxoid stroma

Myxopapillary ependymoma
Chordoma
Peripheral nerve sheath tumor
Metastases

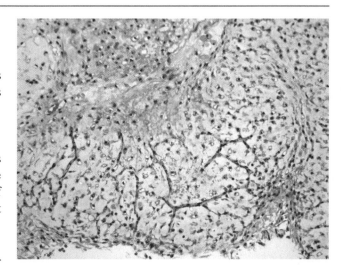

Fig. 5C.9 Histology – chondrosarcoma – chondroid background with small nuclei in lacunes

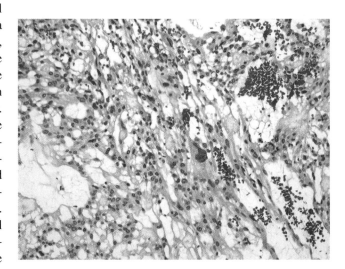

Fig. 5C.10 Histology – myxopapillary ependymoma – microcystic, possibly myxoid tumor with long thin processes and generally small round nuclei, but an occasional large hyperchromatic nucleus

Differential Diagnosis: Myxopapillary Ependymoma

One of the sites for chordoma is sacrum which is very close to the typical location for the myxopapillary variant of ependymoma in the filum/cauda equina. Like chordoma, the myxopapillary ependymoma has a myxoid and cystic background (Fig. 5C.10), but the ependymoma has perivascular pseudorosettes and the cells have processes.

Differential Diagnosis: Metastatic Carcinoma

Mucinous carcinomas can be mistaken for myxoid lesions like chordomas. The cords of eosinophilic cells in chordoma are similar to epithelial rows of cells in some other tumors. Clear cell tumors metastatic to bone may be mistaken for chordoma, but at closer inspection have clear cytoplasm rather than multiple vacuoles within the cytoplasm. Metastatic renal cell carcinoma may show its tendency to hemorrhage (Fig. 5C.11). In comparison to carcinomas, chordomas generally show only minimal pleomorphism, and few mitoses, with no necrosis.

Differential Diagnosis: Chordoid Meningioma

Obviously, from the name, the chordoid subtype of meningioma has similarities to chordoma. When it occurs along the skull base it enters into the differential and may invade or make bone (Fig. 5C.12). The nuclei are still those of meningioma (round to oval with pseudoinclusions).

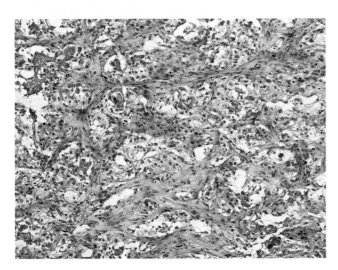

Fig. 5C.11 Histology – metastatic renal cell carcinoma – nests of cells with clear cytoplasm, hemosiderin-laden macrophages, and fibrosis

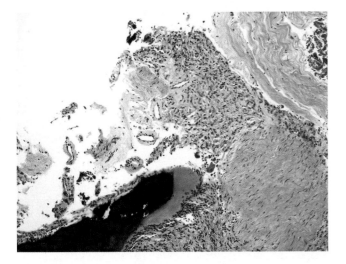

Fig. 5C.12 Histology – chordoid meningioma – myxoid tumor invading bone

Cautions

- Location and scan characteristics narrow the differential considerably.
- Myxoid material often requires overstaining to show up very well.

Bibliography

Chordoma

1. Chopra S, Frank SJ, Gu M. Cytologic diagnosis of chordoma in a peritoneal effusion: a case report. Acta Cytol. 2010;54(3):341–4.
2. Köybaşioğlu F, Simşek GG, Onal BU, Han U, Adabağ A. Oropharyngeal chordoma diagnosed by fine needle aspiration: a case report. Acta Cytol. 2005;49(2):173–6.
3. Layfield LJ. Cytologic differential diagnosis of myxoid and mucinous neoplasms of the sacrum and parasacral soft tissues. Diagn Cytopathol. 2003;28(5):264–71.
4. Kay PA, Nascimento AG, Unni KK, Salomão DR. Chordoma. Cytomorphologic findings in 14 cases diagnosed by fine needle aspiration. Acta Cytol. 2003;47(2):202–8.
5. Chivukula M, Rao R, Macchi J, Ghazala F, Rao RN, Komorowski R, Shidham VB. FNAB cytology of chordoma masquerading as adenocarcinoma: case report. Diagn Cytopathol. 2002;26(5):306–9.
6. Bouvier D, Raghuveer CV. Aspiration cytology of metastatic chordoma to the orbit. Am J Ophthalmol. 2001;131(2):279–80.
7. Crapanzano JP, Ali SZ, Ginsberg MS, Zakowski MF. Chordoma: a cytologic study with histologic and radiologic correlation. Cancer. 2001;93(1):40–51.
8. Ng WK, Tang V. Crush preparation findings of "sarcomatoid" chordoma of the sacrum: report of a case with histologic, immunohistochemical, and ultrastructural correlation. Diagn Cytopathol. 2001;25(6):406–10.

Case 5D
A 23-Year-Old Female with Nasal Congestion and Forehead Pain

Cynthia T. Welsh

Clinical History

- 23-year-old female
- Constant left-sided nasal congestion and facial pain
- No relief with antibiotics
- Exam:
  - Limitation of left eye lateral gaze

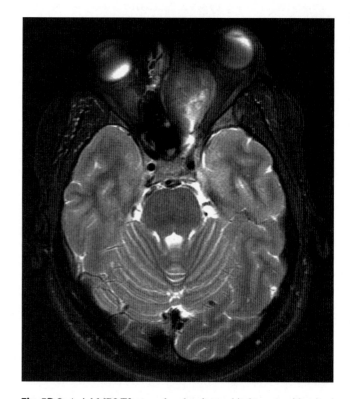

Fig. 5D.2 Axial MRI T2 – nasal and or intraorbital tumor with mixed T2 signal

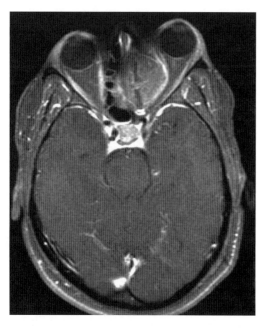

Fig. 5D.1 Axial MRI T1 post-contrast – nasal and or intraorbital tumor compressing optic nerve

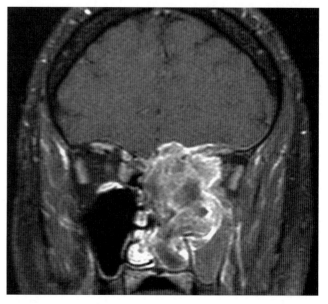

Fig. 5D.3 Coronal MRI T1 post-contrast – heterogeneously enhancing intraorbital and nasal tumor involving the nasal septum and infiltrating through dura into the subdural space inferior to frontal lobe

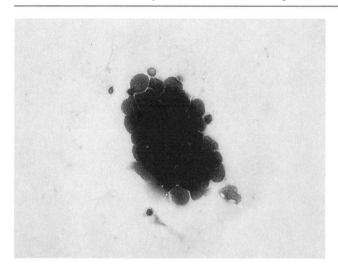

Fig. 5D.4 Smear (DQ stain high magnification) – group of small nuclei with little cytoplasm, little pleomorphism, and with nuclear molding

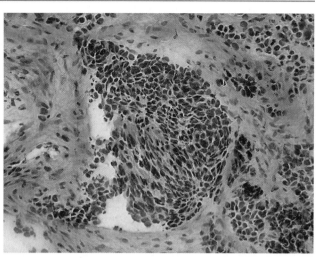

Fig. 5D.6 Frozen section (H&E stain high magnification) – nests of small cells with little cytoplasm and nuclear molding

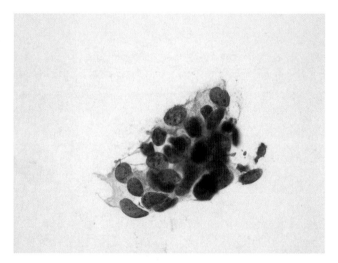

Fig. 5D.5 Smear (H&E stain high magnification) – oval to carrot-shaped nuclei with fine chromatin and minute nucleoli; cytoplasm is scarce

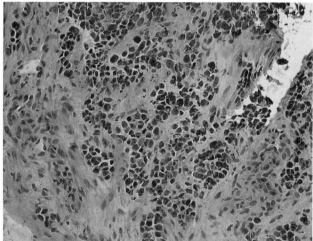

Fig. 5D.7 Frozen section (H&E stain high magnification) – somewhat greater pleomorphism than seen in other areas

What Is Your Diagnosis?

Figure Discussion

Scans

Lesions centered on the roof of the nasopharynx tend to be olfactory neuroblastomas (ONB). The center of the lesion in this case is not as midline as most ONB. The enhancement pattern is heterogeneous (Figs. 5D.1–5D.3).

Pathology

These are small round blue cells without much cytoplasm and variable pleomorphism, that crush easily. The cells not crushed in the tissue sections show mostly round nuclei with some nucleoli, and some molding. There is also fibrosis and single cell death on tissue sections (Figs. 5D.4–5D.7).

Diagnosis: Olfactory Neuroblastoma

Esthesioneuroblastoma (olfactory neuroblastoma) is a midline neoplasm centered on the cribriform plate which causes obstructive symptoms and bleeding, with pain being less common. Either CT or MRI can demonstrate the location, but CT shows the calcifications (if present) better, as well as the bone destruction. The tumors eventually mushroom into the cranium where the differential can include primary and metastatic bone and dural tumors. The tumors are variable depending on grade, and range from sheets or nests of fairly monotonous small round cells to necrotic, pleomorphic, highly proliferative neoplasms. They may show the anuclear process-filled areas (Homer Wright rosettes) that other tumors with small cells and neuronal tendencies have. The cells have scant cytoplasm, and nuclei with "salt and pepper" chromatin.

Differential Diagnosis: Plasma Cell Dyscrasia

The location can be similar for both tumors. Plasma cells can make nests and cords, and be fairly monotonous appearing similar to ONB. The level of necrosis is generally higher in ONB. Plasma cells become less recognizable as they become more immature, but tend to have eccentric nuclei (Fig. 5D.8) with chromatin clumping (perhaps a clock face), golgi "Hoffs," and scattered binucleate cells.

Differential Diagnosis Pituitary Adenoma

The center of the lesion varies somewhat between these two tumors; there should not be tumor in the sella with an ONB. Sheets of cells may appear in either tumor. Zones of necrosis may be seen in adenomas which have infarcted, but single cell apoptosis/karyorrhexis is unusual. Mitoses are usually few if any. Little pleomorphism is present in adenomas (Fig. 5D.9).

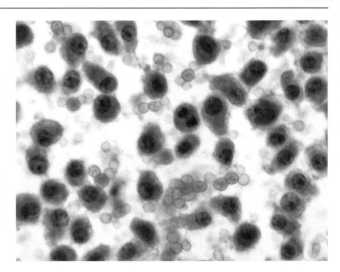

Fig. 5D.8 Touch preparation – myeloma – eccentric round nuclei with chromatin clumping (which tends to be along nuclear membrane – "clockface") and nucleoli. Scattered binucleate cells and perinuclear cytoplasmic clearing (Hoffs). The cytoplasm is amphophilic (*purple*) because both the eosin (protein) and hematoxylin (nucleic acid) stains the cytoplasm

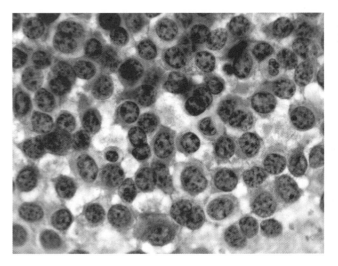

Fig. 5D.9 Touch preparation – pituitary adenoma – single cells with eccentric round monotonous nuclei with chromatin clumping and nucleoli. Occasional binucleate cells

Differential Diagnosis: Invasion from the Paranasal Sinuses/Nasopharynx

Tumors from the paranasal sinuses, nasopharynx, salivary glands, and other areas of the face may invade the cranium. Some (such as adenoid cystic carcinoma) particularly have a tendency to do this, often by way of the cranial nerves (Fig. 5D.10) and can have a nonspecific resemblance to many tumors including ONB (Fig. 5D.11). Sinonasal carcinomas

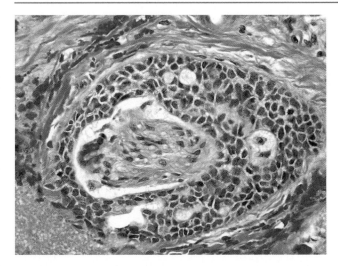

Fig. 5D.10 Histology – adenoid cystic carcinoma – perineural spread of apparently epithelial tumor with vacuolated cytoplasm

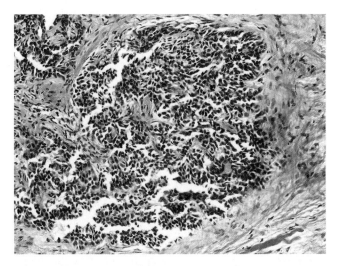

Fig. 5D.11 Histology – adenoid cystic carcinoma – nests of fairly small bland nuclei with no specific features

are anaplastic large cell tumors with prominent necrosis and are often clearly epithelial. Melanomas from the skin or mucosa may invade into the cribriform plate/base of skull. Depending on the cell type, the cells will generally be more spindled or larger with prominent nucleoli, unlike ONB.

Cautions

Knowing the location from the scans makes the differential much narrower than it would be otherwise. Many of these tumors are very similar on frozen sections.

Bibliography

Olfactory Neuroblastoma

1. Bellizzi AM, Bourne TD, Mills SE, Stelow EB. The cytologic features of sinonasal undifferentiated carcinoma and olfactory neuroblastoma. Am J Clin Pathol. 2008;129(3):367–76.
2. Mahooti S, Wakely PE Jr. Cytopathologic features of olfactory neuroblastoma. Cancer. 2006;108(2):86–92.
3. Chung J, Park ST, Jang J. Fine needle aspiration cytology of metastatic olfactory neuroblastoma: a case report. Acta Cytol. 2002;46(1): 40–5.
4. Perez-Ordonez B, Caruana SM, Huvos AG, Shah JP. Small cell neuroendocrine carcinoma of the nasal cavity and paranasal sinuses. Hum Pathol. 1998;29(8):826–32.
5. Collins BT, Cramer HM, Hearn SA. Fine needle aspiration cytology of metastatic olfactory neuroblastoma. Acta Cytol. 1997;41(3): 802–10.

Case 5E
An 18-Year-Old Female with Headache

Cynthia T. Welsh

Clinical History

- 18-year-old pregnant female
- Severe headache
- History of sickle cell trait
- Normal neurologic exam

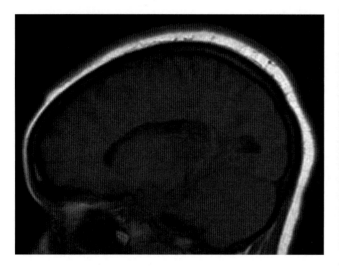

Fig. 5E.1 Sagittal MRI T1 precontrast – posterior midline mass possibly in lateral ventricle

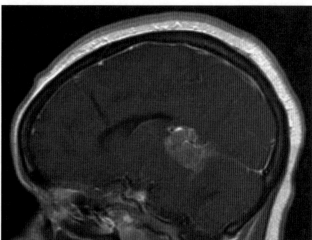

Fig. 5E.2 Sagittal MRI T1 postcontrast – enhancing mass in thalamus/pineal area

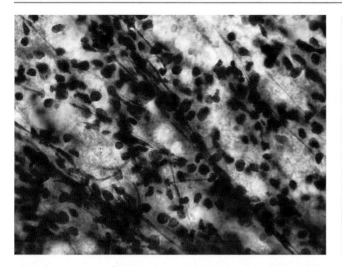

Fig. 5E.3 Smear (H&E stain high magnification) – small round nuclei with some variation in nuclear size, coarse chromatin, and distinct nuclear membrane

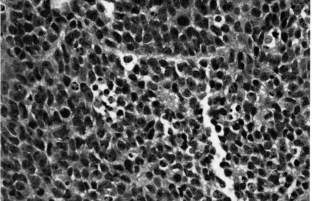

Fig. 5E.5 Frozen section (H&E stain high magnification) – closer view of discohesive cells, single cell death, and incomplete rings of nuclei around relatively anuclear areas

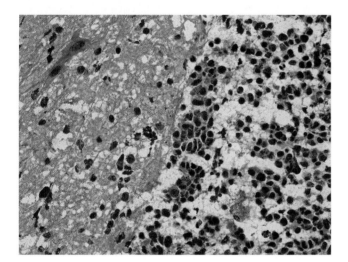

Fig. 5E.4 Frozen section (H&E stain high magnification) – small cells with little cytoplasm mainly abutting brain, but also probably showing single cell infiltration

What Is Your Diagnosis?

Figure Discussion

Scans

It can be difficult, especially with a large tumor to tell the origin. Looking at different views helps tell that this tumor is centered in the pineal and the contrast makes it easier to see (Figs. 5E.1–5E.2).

Pathology

Many different types of small round blue cell tumors (SRBCTs) are seen in brain, the differential depends on age and location. The rosettes with central anuclear areas of neuropil seen here place the differential in the category of tumors with neuroblastic tendencies. Also seen are discohesive cells with small round nuclei, some variation in nuclear size, coarse chromatin, distinct nuclear membranes, and single cell death (Figs. 5E.3–5E.5).

Diagnosis: Pineoblastoma

Tumors in the pineal region in childhood tend to be pineoblastomas or germ cell tumors. In an adult, they are more often pineocytomas, where the differential diagnosis is cystic and gliotic "normal" pineal. Pineoblastomas are seldom very cystic and enhance on scans. Craniospinal dissemination is common. They have the small neuroblastic type (Homer Wright) rosettes (Table 5E.1), which may show up on a smear where they haven't been pulled apart, and will be apparent (but perhaps subtle) on frozen section. These are SRBCTs (Table 5E.2) with high cellularity, necrosis, and numerous mitoses. On either smears or sections, these cells have little cytoplasm and hyperchromatic nuclei. Intraoperatively, diagnosis is most often "SRBCT of childhood."

Differential Diagnosis: Normal Pineal/Pineal Cyst

The normal pineal has cells very similar to the pineocytoma, and both have cystic tendencies, but normal pineal has a lobular pattern (Fig. 5E.6). These can be difficult to separate out

Table 5E.1 Neuronal/neuroblastic rosettes

Medulloblastoma
Central PNET
Pineoblastoma
Pineocytoma
Neurocytoma
Rosetted glioneuronal tumor
Peripheral neuroblastoma
Ewing sarcoma/peripheral PNET
Esthesioneuroblastoma

Table 5E.2 Small cell neoplasms

Medulloblastoma
PNETs (ependymoblastoma, cerebral neuroblastoma)
Small cell metastases
Lymphoma
Small cell glioblastoma Pineoblastoma
Germinoma
Rhabdomyosarcoma
Ewing sarcoma
Esthesioneuroblastoma
SNUC (sinonasal undifferentiated carcinoma)

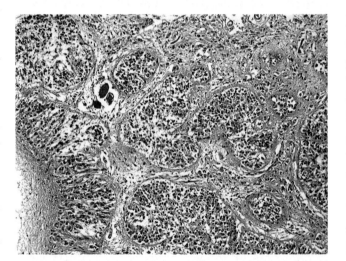

Fig. 5E.6 Histology – normal adult pineal – nested cells with a cyst in the central glial part of the pineal (lower left corner of the figure) which is very common in adult pineal

even on permanent sections, much less on frozen sections. Pineoblastoma nuclei on the other hand are larger than normal cells, more pleomorphic, very mitotically active, and show necrosis (including single cell necrosis).

Differential Diagnosis: Medulloblastoma

It may be difficult sometimes on scans to tell where a large tumor is centered. Medulloblastoma, like pineoblastoma, is a very cellular tumor with a high nuclear to cytoplasmic ratio (Fig. 5E.7). Either may demonstrate Homer Wright type rosettes. Both have a tendency toward leptomeningeal spread. The pineal recess is actually close enough to the posterior fossa for the differential to sometimes be in doubt. Either one intraoperatively can be called just "SRBCT of childhood."

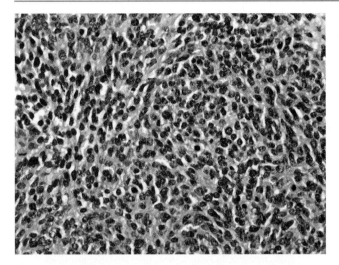

Fig. 5E.7 Histology – medulloblastoma – sheets of small round blue cells with mitoses, single cell death, and neuroblastic rosettes

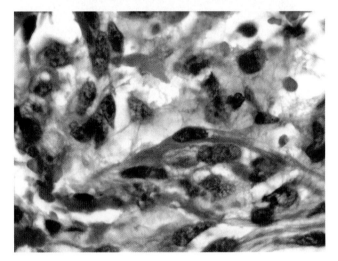

Fig. 5E.8 Histology – rhabdomyosarcoma – large vesicular nuclei with prominent nucleoli and in general little cytoplasm, but occasional "strap" cells

Differential Diagnosis: Other Metastatic/Primary Small Round Blue Cell Tumors

Ewing's sarcoma and neuroblastoma metastasize to skull, many tumors (particularly leukemias and lymphomas) can metastasize to leptomeninges/dura, and even SRBCTs of childhood such as rhabdomyosarcoma can occur as a primary (Fig. 5E.8) or metastatic tumor in leptomeninges/dura.

Differential Diagnosis: Germ Cell Neoplasm

Intracranial germ cell neoplasms occur in the midline, generally in the pituitary or pineal regions. Because of this they enter the differential in those regions, especially in the

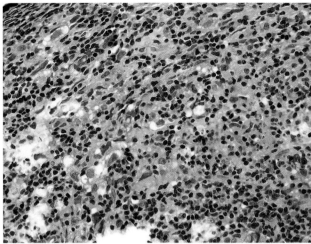

Fig. 5E.9 Histology – germinoma – lymphocytic background and sprinkled large cells with eosinophilic or vacuolated cytoplasm and large nuclei with occasional prominent nucleoli

pediatric age group. The more diffuse type with sheets of cells such as the germinoma (Fig. 5E.9) or embryonal carcinoma are most likely to be mistaken for pineoblastoma.

Cautions

Differential with SRBCT depends to a large extent on age, location, and history.

Bibliography

Pineoblastoma

1. Ghosal N, Furtado SV, Hegde AS. Rosette forming glioneuronal tumor pineal gland and tectum: An intraoperative diagnosis on smear preparation. Diagn Cytopathol. 2009;38(8):590–3.
2. Shimada K, Nakamura M, Kuga Y, Taomoto K, Ohnishi H, Konishi N. Cytologic feature by squash preparation of pineal parenchyma tumor of intermediate differentiation. Diagn Cytopathol. 2008;36(10):749–53.
3. Buccoliero AM, Sardi I, Castiglione F, Mussa F, Giordano F, Genitori L, Taddei GL. Pineal germinoma morphological features in a liquid-based cerebrospinal fluid sample. Diagn Cytopathol. 2008;36(9):645–6.
4. Geramizadeh B, Daneshbood Y, Karimi M. Cytology of brain metastasis of yolk sac tumor. Acta Cytol. 2005;49(1):110–1.
5. Parwani AV, Baisden BL, Erozan YS, Burger PC, Ali SZ. Pineal gland lesions: a cytopathologic study of 20 specimens. Cancer. 2005;105(2):80–6.
6. Hoda RS, Hoda SA, Reuter VE. Intraoperative touch-imprint cytology of germ cell neoplasms. Diagn Cytopathol. 1996;14(4):393–4.
7. Ng HK. Cytologic diagnosis of intracranial germinomas in smear preparations. Acta Cytol. 1995;39(4):693–7.

Case 5F
A 11-Year-Old Male with Headache, Nausea, Vomiting

Cynthia T. Welsh

Clinical History

- 11-year-old male
- History of migraines × 2 years
- Headache × 6 days, vomiting × 2 days
- Normal neurologic exam

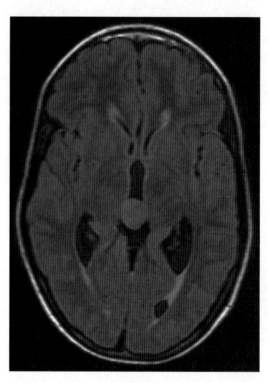

Fig. 5F.2 Axial MRI T2 FLAIR – slightly bright posterior third ventricle mass

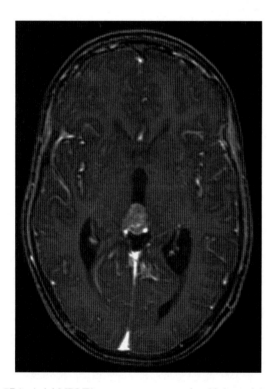

Fig. 5F.1 Axial MRI T1 postcontrast – posterior third ventricle mass which enhances

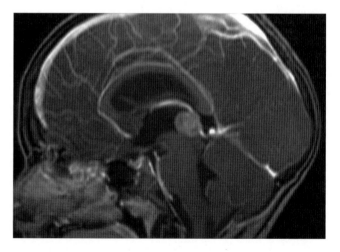

Fig. 5F.3 Sagittal MRI T1 postcontrast – enhancing pineal mass

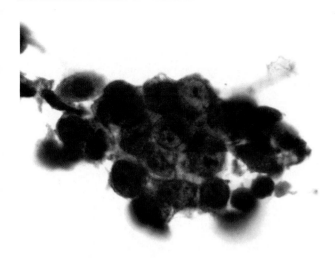

Fig. 5F.4 Smear (H&E stain high magnification) – large cells with multiple chromocenters and small amounts of eosinophilic cytoplasm, and smaller nuclei with scant cytoplasm

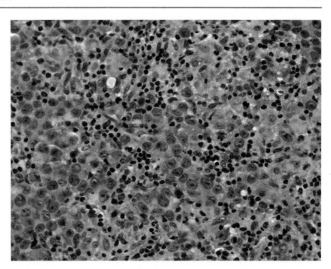

Fig. 5F.6 Frozen section (H&E stain high magnification) – large cells with red macronucleoli and a second smaller cell population

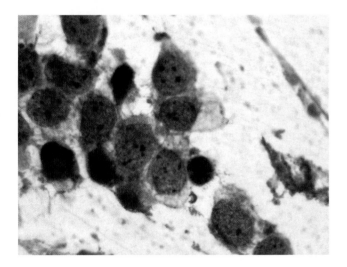

Fig. 5F.5 Smear (H&E stain high magnification) – large cells with multiple chromocenters and small amounts of eosinophilic cytoplasm, and rare smaller nuclei with scant cytoplasm

What Is Your Diagnosis?

Figure Discussion

Scans

Pineal region tumors can be difficult to localize when very large, but this tumor is small enough that a posterior third ventricle location is more obvious. The tumor enhances well (Figs. 5F.1–5F.3).

Pathology

Tumor cells with little cytoplasm in the CNS in children tend to be primary neuronal tumors, but in this case are something else. There are two cell populations in both smears and sections. The smaller cells are lymphocytes. The large cells are not very pleomorphic, with lots of cytoplasm, and large nuclei with large nucleoli (Figs. 5F.4–5F.6).

Diagnosis: Germ Cell Tumor

Germ cell tumors in the CNS are most often seen in the sellar and pineal areas in children. The specific types seen vary by age, gender, and location. They include all the types seen elsewhere including mature or immature teratomas, embryonal, yolk sac, germinoma, and choriocarcinoma.

Some of these tumors elicit a very robust granulomatous reaction, so that non-neoplastic lesions such as sarcoid (Fig. 5F.7) can be in the differential. Similarly, Langerhans cell histiocytosis (LCH) may be considered sometimes (Fig. 5F.8). The germ cell tumor in this case is a germinoma, which characteristically has large cells with abundant cytoplasm and large (sometimes vesicular) nuclei with prominent nucleoli admixed with lymphocytes. The cytoplasm of the large cells may appear clear or eosinophilic. Human chori-

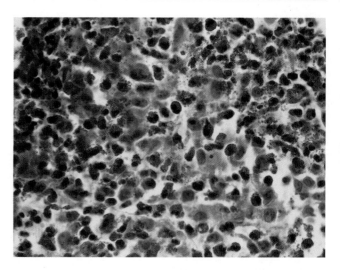

Fig. 5F.8 Histology – LCH – background eosinophils and a second population of large cells with large nuclei and fairly prominent nucleoli

onic gonadotropin (HCG) levels may be mildly elevated without there being a choriocarcinoma component because of scattered syncytiotrophoblastic cells.

Differential Diagnosis: Pineoblastoma/Medulloblastoma

Along the base of the skull, tumors in children are more often medulloblastoma or pineoblastoma (depending on location) than germ cell tumors. Both SRBCTs can be very similar in appearance, with the so-called small round cell tumor of childhood appearance (Fig. 5F.9) seen in this medulloblastoma or Homer Wright rosettes may be apparent leading one to recognize the neuronal predilection of the tumor (Fig. 5F.10) as in this pineoblastoma. Neither have the lymphoid background of the germinoma.

Differential Diagnosis: Pituitary

Pituitary adenomas are unusual in children but do occur, and are in one of the areas where germ cell tumors can be also seen (the sella). The cells of a pituitary adenoma are fairly small, and monotonous. They are often binucleate with eccentric nuclei (Fig. 5F.11). They generally have few mitoses and little pleomorphism. While they have many architectural patterns, the cells are less changeable.

Differential Diagnosis: Metastatic Tumors

Yolk sac tumors in particular can be mimicked by carcinomas. These are fortunately rarely metastatic to the central nervous system in children. Lymphoma and leukemia in the

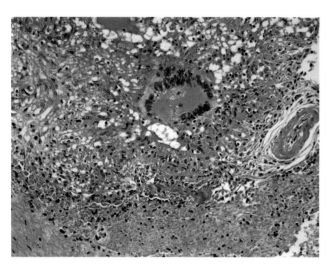

Fig. 5F.7 Histology – sarcoid – multinucleated giant cell with an "asteroid" body and adjacent palisading histiocytes and almost no lymphocytes

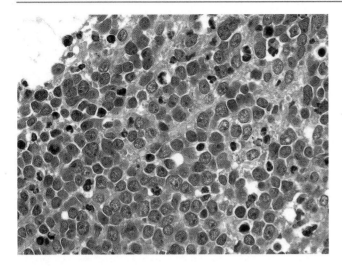

Fig. 5F.9 Histology – anaplastic/large cell medulloblastoma – mostly large round nuclei with some molding and prominent nucleoli, little cytoplasm, neuronal rosettes, and prominent single cell death

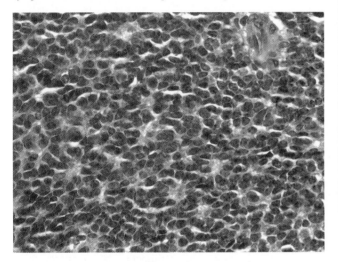

Fig. 5F.10 Histology – pineoblastoma – very cellular tumor with little cytoplasm, round to oval nuclei, and neuronal rosettes

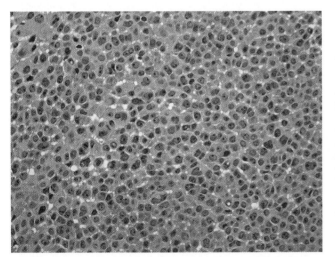

Fig. 5F.11 Histology – pituitary adenoma – sheets of monotonous cells with eosinophilic cytoplasm, mostly round nuclei with fine pale chromatin, and fairly prominent nucleoli. Occasional binucleate cells are present

leptomeninges/dura are among the small round blue cell tumors of childhood that may mimic germ cell tumors, especially germinoma. Ewing's sarcoma (Fig. 5F.12) or neuroblastoma metastatic to the skullbase may enter into the differential.

Differential Diagnosis: Ependymoma

Germ cell tumors can grow so large in children that they often can appear ventricular at least in part and enter the differential for ependymoma. Ependymomas have perivascular pseudorosettes (Fig. 5F.13), which are not seen in germ cell tumors (except the rare teratoma with an ependymoma in it).

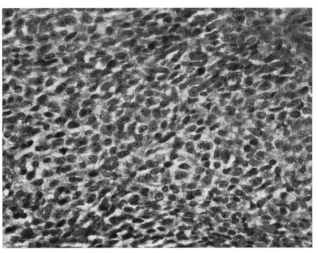

Fig. 5F.12 Histology – Ewing's sarcoma – sheets of cells with vacuolated cytoplasm and somewhat vesicular nuclei with nucleoli

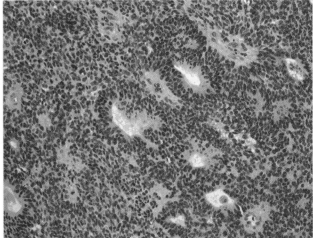

Fig. 5F.13 Histology – ependymoma – cellular, mitotically active tumor with perivascular pseudorosettes and true rosettes

Cautions

- HCG levels may be elevated in germinoma without choriocarcinoma.
- A granulomatous reaction may obscure germ cell tumor morphology.

Bibliography

Germ Cell Tumor

1. Ohta Y, Suzuki T, Tonoike T, Hamatani S, Ohike N, Shiokawa A, Kushima M, Ota H. Two cases of intracranial germinoma showing a cell arrangement mimicking carcinoma. Diagn Cytopathol. 2010; 38(2):132–6.
2. Ghosal N, Furtado SV, Hegde AS. Rosette forming glioneuronal tumor pineal gland and tectum: an intraoperative diagnosis on smear preparation. Diagn Cytopathol. 2009;38(8):590–3.
3. Shimada K, Nakamura M, Kuga Y, Taomoto K, Ohnishi H, Konishi N. Cytologic feature by squash preparation of pineal parenchyma tumor of intermediate differentiation. Diagn Cytopathol. 2008; 36(10):749–53.
4. Buccoliero AM, Sardi I, Castiglione F, Mussa F, Giordano F, Genitori L, Taddei GL. Pineal germinoma morphological features in a liquid-based cerebrospinal fluid sample. Diagn Cytopathol. 2008;36(9): 645–6.
5. Geramizadeh B, Daneshbood Y, Karimi M. Cytology of brain metastasis of yolk sac tumor. Acta Cytol. 2005;49(1):110–1.
6. Parwani AV, Baisden BL, Erozan YS, Burger PC, Ali SZ. Pineal gland lesions: a cytopathologic study of 20 specimens. Cancer. 2005;105(2):80–6.
7. Loo CK, Freeman B, Stanford D, Gune S. Cytologic findings in a fetal intracranial teratoma. A case report. Acta Cytol. 2001; 45(2):227–32.
8. Hoda RS, Hoda SA, Reuter VE. Intraoperative touch-imprint cytology of germ cell neoplasms. Diagn Cytopathol. 1996;14(4): 393–4.
9. Ng HK. Cytologic diagnosis of intracranial germinomas in smear preparations. Acta Cytol. 1995;39(4):693–7.

The Spinal Neoplasm in an Adult

6

Case 6A:
A 44-Year-Old Male with Leg and Back Pain

Cynthia T. Welsh

Clinical History

- 44-year-old male
- Leg and back pain
- Negative neurologic exam

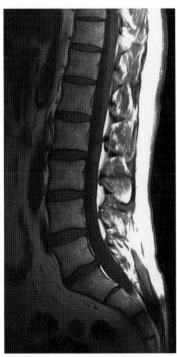

Fig. 6A.1 Sagittal MRI T1 precontrast – nodular, well-circumscribed lesion

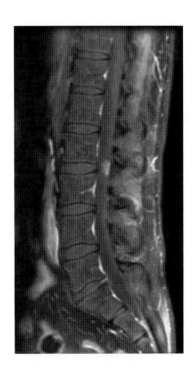

Fig. 6A.2 Sagittal MRI T1 postcontrast – brightly enhancing

C.T. Welsh (ed.), *Intra-Operative Neuropathology for the Non-Neuropathologist: A Case-Based Approach*,
DOI 10.1007/978-1-4419-1167-4_6, © Springer Science+Business Media, LLC 2012

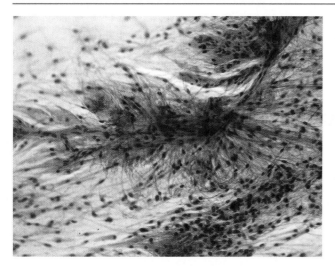

Fig. 6A.3 Smear (H&E stain low magnification) – cells "feather" away from vessels

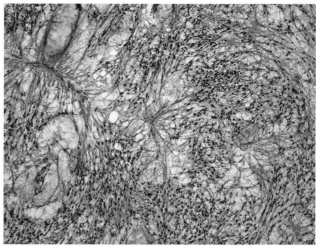

Fig. 6A.4 Frozen section (H&E stain low magnification) – myxoid change and perivascular pseudorosettes

What Is Your Diagnosis?

Figure Discussion

Scans

The sagittal MRI pre- and postcontrast scans show a small lumbar spine lesion which enhances well demonstrating how circumscribed it is (Figs. 6A.1–6A.2).

Pathology

There is myxoid change, and ependymal perivascular pseudorosettes are apparent on both histology and smears. The nuclei are oval and have delicate chromatin. The processes indicate this is a glial tumor, and the association with the vessels makes it ependymal (Figs. 6A.3–6A.4).

Diagnosis: Myxopapillary Ependymoma

Tumors at the cauda equina/filum terminale often present with "cauda equina" syndrome (bowel/bladder problems, and leg weakness) in addition to back pain. This is the most common location for the myxopapillary variant of ependymoma. The tumors are more common in males, and the patients are often young (teen to young adult). Myxopapillary ependymomas enhance well and are usually discrete, encapsulated masses. On sections they have lobules. They smear well, and show pseudorosettes like other ependymomas on both smears and sections, with the addition of myxoid areas (Table 6A.1) around the vessels, which are typically (but not always) hyalinized (Fig. 6A.5). The myxoid areas may not show up well unless the sections are well stained. Unfortunately, myxopapillary ependymomas frequently also do not appear particularly papillary, as in this case. These cells have bland oval nuclei and processes. You don't want to intra-operatively just say ependymoma, but rather myxopapillary ependymoma, because this subtype is WHO grade 1 without the treatment implications attached to the other ependymomas.

Differential Diagnosis: Chordoma

The area where myxopapillary ependymomas usually occur is adjacent to one of the sites where chordomas are common, the sacrum. Both have a myxoid background, lobules of cells, and cystic change. Knowing that the tumor is centered in the sacrum makes it more likely chordoma. Recognizing

Table 6A.1 Myxoid stroma

Myxopapillary ependymoma
Chordoma
Peripheral nerve sheath tumor
Metastases

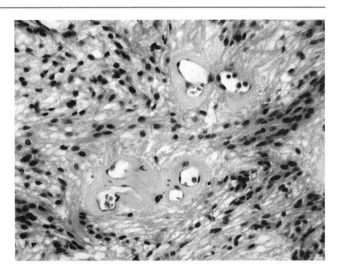

Fig. 6A.5 Histology – myxopapillary ependymoma – hyalinized vessels with surrounding loose areas around which nuclei congregate

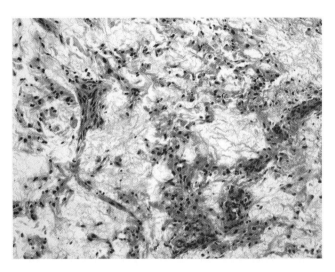

Fig. 6A.6 Histology – chordoma – cords of eosinophilic cells in a myxoid matrix

the cords of cells with eosinophilic cytoplasm in the myxoid background (Fig. 6A.6) or the foamy physaliferous cells will clinch the diagnosis.

Differential Diagnosis: Peripheral Nerve Sheath Tumor

Schwannomas and neurofibromas occur at the lower portions of the cord/cauda equina also. Both can have a loose myxoid appearance and long spindled cells similar to myxopapillary ependymoma. The vessels in schwannomas are hyalinized like the ones in the myxopapillary ependymoma. The perivascular pseudorosettes and lobular architecture (possibly

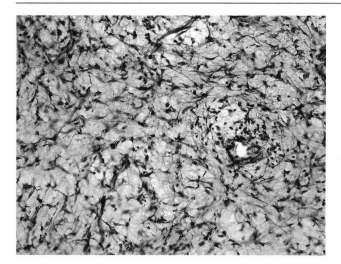

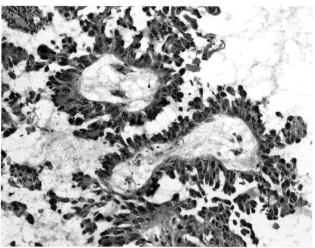

Fig. 6A.7 Histology – schwannoma – spindle nuclei, processes, loose areas which could be frozen artifact, and occasional large hyperchromatic nuclei

Fig. 6A.8 Histology – metastatic tumor – papillary architecture covered with multiple layers of cells with hyperchromatic, irregular nuclei and some nucleoli

papillary) of the myxopapillary ependymoma will not be present in schwannoma. Peripheral nerve sheath tumors do not smear well, unlike ependymomas. The appearance on frozen sections will often be bland spindle cells (Fig. 6A.7), but sometimes the biphasic nature will be apparent, and you may even have Verocay bodies.

Differential Diagnosis: Papillary/Mucinous Metastatic Neoplasms

Tumors more often metastasize to vertebral column, dura, or leptomeninges than to the spinal cord itself. Myxoid material and mucin can look very similar, especially on frozen sections. The history of a systemic carcinoma should help bring it into the differential. Looking at the morphology of the cells in the material will help sort out whether you are looking at something malignant and metastatic or the histologically benign myxopapillary ependymoma. Papillary metastatic tumors are usually necrotic and mitotically active, unlike myxopapillary ependymomas. They generally have fibrovascular cores surrounded by tumor cells (Fig. 6A.8) as opposed to the pseudorosette.

Cautions

Myxopapillary ependymoma may not be papillary and the myxoid background may require overstaining to make it show up very well.

References

Myxopapillary Ependymoma

1. Bradly DP, Reddy VB, Cochran E, Gattuso P. Comparison of cytological features of myxopapillary ependymomas on crush preparations. Diagn Cytopathol. 2009;37(8):607–12.
2. Takei H, Kosarac O, Powell SZ. Cytomorphologic features of myxopapillary ependymoma: a review of 13 cases. Acta Cytol. 2009; 53(3):297–302.
3. Layfield LJ. Cytologic differential diagnosis of myxoid and mucinous neoplasms of the sacrum and parasacral soft tissues. Diagn Cytopathol. 2003;28(5):264–71.
4. Kulesza P, Tihan T, Ali SZ. Myxopapillary ependymoma: cytomorphologic characteristics and differential diagnosis. Diagn Cytopathol. 2002;26(4):247–50.
5. Ortega L, Jiménez-Heffernan JA, Sanz E, Ortega P. Squash cytology of intradural myxopapillary ependymoma. Acta Cytol. 2002;46(2):428–30.
6. Bardales RH, Porter MC, Sawyer JR, Mrak RE, Stanley MW. Metastatic myxopapillary ependymoma: report of a case with fine-needle aspiration findings. Diagn Cytopathol. 1994;10(1):47–53.

Case 6B:
A 36-Year-Old Male with Leg Weakness and History of Neurofibromatosis 1 (NF1)

Cynthia T. Welsh

Clinical History

- 36-year-old male
- Increasing difficulty walking
- History of NF1
- Multiple previous spinal surgeries
- Exam:
  - Can't stand without support
  - Sensory level above umbilicus
  - Increased reflexes lower extremities

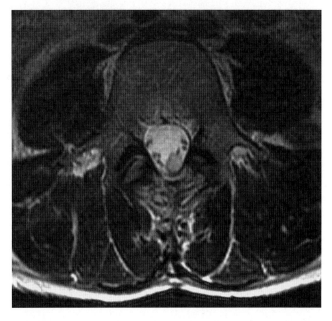

Fig. 6B.2 Axial MRI T2 – CSF is brighter than the mass, the dark areas are spinal nerves

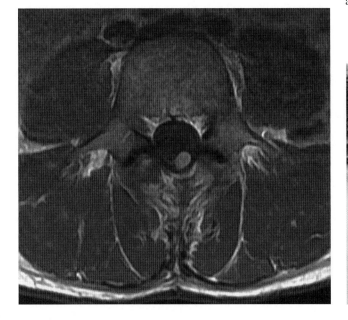

Fig. 6B.1 Axial MRI T1 postcontrast – small well-circumscribed homogeneously contrast enhancing mass posterior to spinal cord

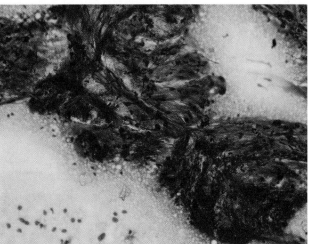

Fig. 6B.3 Smear (DQ stain low magnification) – the tissue does not smear well; in the effort to squash/smear it, the nuclei have also been smeared

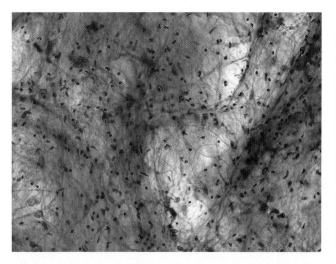

Fig. 6B.4 Smear (H&E stain low magnification) – tissue fragments are not very cellular and not finely fibrillary/vacuolated

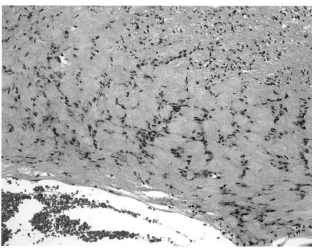

Fig. 6B.6 Frozen section (H&E stain low magnification) – palisading nuclei

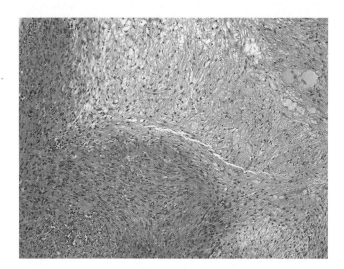

Fig. 6B.5 Frozen section (H&E stain low magnification) – biphasic architecture

What Is Your Diagnosis?

Figure Discussion

Scans

Small round well-circumscribed extra-axial (outside spinal cord) lesion, posterior to and compressing cord, which enhances (Figs. 6B.1–6B.2).

Pathology

The smears show clumps of tissue that didn't smear well and quite a bit of variation in nuclear size and shape. Some larger cells in the background almost appear neuronal. The tissue sections show a biphasic pattern with loose focally microcystic areas (Antoni B) and the higher magnification of a denser area (Antoni A) shows cells in palisades along relatively anuclear areas (Verocay bodies) (Figs. 6B.3–6B.6).

Diagnosis: Schwannoma

Extra-axial intradural neoplasms of the spinal canal may be peripheral nerve sheath, meningeal, or metastatic. Ependymomas and paragangliomas also can occur there. Typically, benign peripheral nerve sheath tumors (BPNST), particularly schwannomas, are sporadic. Multiple schwannomas suggest either NF2 or schwannomatosis. Most spinal schwannomas are seen in adults. Just as cerebellopontine angle schwannomas are usually on the vestibular division of cranial nerve eight, spinal schwannomas occur most often on sensory nerve roots, so they tend to be posterior to the cord, as in this case. Schwannomas are often cystic, they enhance well, and the spinal ones may erode bone and/or have a dumbbell shape from crawling through the neural foramen. This patient had NF1, so clinically was suspected to have a neurofibroma. The diagnosis at intra-operative consultation is very often just "low grade (or benign) peripheral nerve sheath tumor," or spindle cell lesion anyway, depending on the amount of differentiation seen. Schwannomas have thick hyalinized vessel walls with hemosiderin usually scattered nearby as opposed to neurofibromas. If Antoni A (cellular, compact) areas are present with oval to elongated nuclei, then it is a schwannoma. If only the Antoni B loose areas with wavy nuclei are present, it may be either BPNST. Schwannomas are among the benign/low grade tumors (Table 6B.1) which commonly have scattered large, hyperchromatic irregular nuclei.

Table 6B.1 Scattered large irregular hyperchromatic nuclei

Pilocytic astrocytoma
Hemangioblastoma
Meningioma
Schwannoma

Differential Diagnosis: Neurofibroma

Neurofibromas in spinal roots often infiltrate into and expand the ganglion (Fig. 6B.7). The appearance can be similar to a ganglioneuroma. Neurofibromas are virtually inseparable from the loose Antoni B areas of schwannomas. Keep in mind that sampling can be an intra-operative issue with the denser Antoni A areas not appearing until later specimens.

Differential Diagnosis: Meningioma

Meningiomas in the spinal canal have a more decidedly female predominance than even the intracranial ones, so are less likely to enter the differential in a young male. NF1 does not increase his likelihood of having spinal meningiomas either. Meningiomas do not have the predilection for the posterior aspect of the cord that schwannomas do. Neither tumor will squash well, although the meningioma will usually have more cells adhere to the slide than a schwannoma. Whirls of cells, psammoma bodies (Fig. 6B.8), and intranuclear cytoplasmic pseudoinclusions may be seen. The nuclei are more round to slightly oval than the spindled nuclei of schwannoma.

Differential Diagnosis: Myxopapillary Ependymoma

The myxoid background and spindled cells of an ependymoma can be misinterpreted as schwannoma. Myxopapillary ependymomas are most common in the filum/cauda equina, but schwannomas may also occur there, and ependymomas

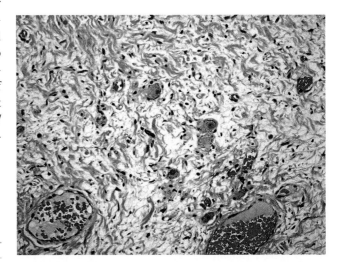

Fig. 6B.7 Histology – neurofibroma – loose tissue with clumps of collagen and small wavy pointed nuclei invading a ganglion with normal ganglion cells some of which have some satellite cells

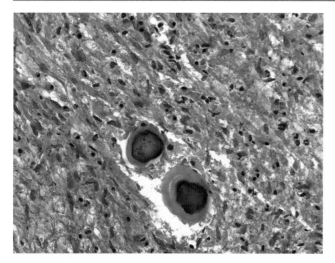

Fig. 6B.8 Histology – meningioma – nondescript tissue with psammoma bodies

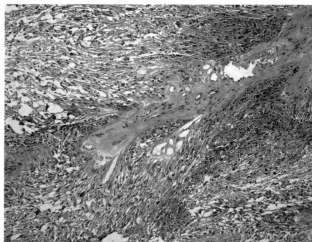

Fig. 6B.10 Histology – pilocytic astrocytoma – hyalinized vessels, long thin "hair-like" processes, and the occasional large dark nucleus

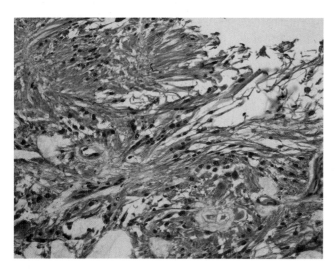

Fig. 6B.9 Histology – myxopapillary ependymoma – long thin processes, a hint of anuclear zones around vessels, and small round to oval nuclei

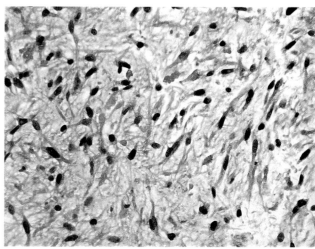

Fig. 6B.11 Smear – pilocytic astrocytoma – spindle nuclei and unipolar to bipolar appearing cytoplasm

can occur at any level. The patient profile is often young male. The symptoms are usually back pain, as with schwannomas. Ependymomas of any type generally smear well. The perivascular arrays (pseudorosettes) of cells (Fig. 6B.9) on either smear or frozen section give away the ependymal nature of this tumor.

Differential Diagnosis: Pilocytic Astrocytoma

Running into one of the rare intraparenchymal schwannomas or not knowing about the extra-axial location of the specimen at which you are looking, may bring pilocytic astrocytoma into the differential. Both are biphasic, have hyalinized vessels (Fig. 6B.10), and may be cystic. Pilocytic astrocytomas of the spinal cord are less common than intracranial ones, but not uncommon. They are more often pediatric no matter what the location. Knowing whether the tumor is in the cord (intra-axial/pilocytic) or outside the cord (extra-axial/schwannoma) is the best place to start with the differential. Pilocytic astrocytomas smear better than schwannomas. Rosenthal fibers and/or granular bodies, if present, help you tell that it is a pilocytic. Hair-like "piloid" bipolar cells may be seen (Fig. 6B.11).

Differential Diagnosis: Ganglioneuroma/Blastoma

Neuroblastoma, ganglioneuroblastoma, and ganglioneuroma occur not just as adrenal masses but also as paraspinal masses which can involve the extradural dural space in addition. Both the cells and the stroma have a range of differentiation which may produce a mature ganglioneuroma. This can be confused with peripheral nerve sheath tumors. Neurofibromas in spinal nerves may invade back up into the ganglia (as in Fig. 6B.7), but those normal ganglion cells have normal satelliting cells around them. The ganglion cells of a ganglioneuroma cluster, and tend toward multinucleation. They often have cytoplasmic vacuoles and do not have normal satellite cells. The ganglioneuroma has a very schwannian stroma (Fig. 6B.12), so if there are no ganglion cells in your intraoperative specimen, you might easily think it a schwannoma. History and scan characteristics may help to narrow your differential. "Spindle cell lesion" may be the most general and applicable frozen diagnosis, and should not alter surgery.

Differential Diagnosis: Malignant Spindle Cell Tumors (Primary or Metastatic)

Hemangiopericytoma (Fig. 6B.13), like meningioma, may enter the differential on scans. These tumors are less common than nerve sheath tumors and meningiomas. The radiologist may see larger feeding vessels entering the tumor, but will most likely consider it probably a meningioma. Hemangiopericytomas smear much better than schwannomas. The cells on smears show distinct cytoplasmic borders and round to oval nuclei, not the elongate nuclei of schwannian tumors. On

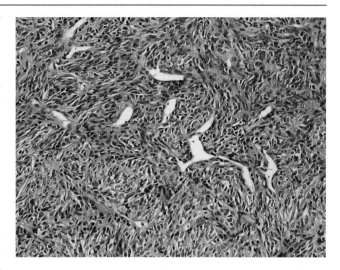

Fig. 6B.13 Histology – hemangiopericytoma – cellular tumor with "staghorn" vessels

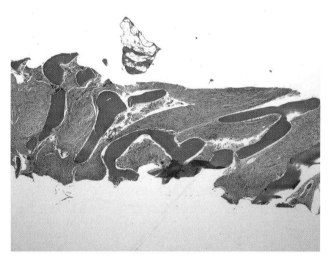

Fig. 6B.14 Histology – metastatic tumor – this core biopsy of bone shows tumor surrounding trabecula of bone

sections, at low power, the first impression will be of the "staghorn" and slit-like vessels. These tumors are cellular (the nuclei often overlap and are randomly oriented). Nuclei are round to oval without much cytoplasm. Metastatic sarcomas often end up in lung or bone, occasionally even skull or vertebral column. Depending on the type of tumor, they may destroy bone or permeate through marrow spaces (Fig. 6B.14).

Cautions

- Verocay-like structures can be seen in leiomyomas.
- Sampling of only the loose Antoni B areas of a schwannoma may make you think it is a neurofibroma.

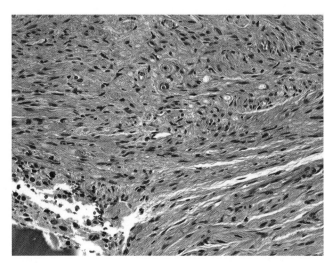

Fig. 6B.12 Histology – ganglioneuroma – within the schwannian background are ganglion cells which have no satellite cells

References

Schwannoma

1. Azarpira N, Torabineghad S, Sepidbakht S, Rakei M, Bagheri MH. Cytologic findings in pigmented melanotic schwannoma: a case report. Acta Cytol. 2009;53(1):113–5.
2. Li S, Ai SZ, Owens C, Kulesza P. Intrapancreatic schwannoma diagnosed by endoscopic ultrasound-guided fine-needle aspiration cytology. Diagn Cytopathol. 2009;37(2):132–5.
3. Klijanienko J, Caillaud JM, Lagacé R. Cytohistologic correlations in schwannomas (neurilemmomas), including "ancient," cellular, and epithelioid variants. Diagn Cytopathol. 2006;34(8): 517–22.
4. Akhtar I, Flowers R, Siddiqi A, Heard K, Baliga M. Fine needle aspiration biopsy of vertebral and paravertebral lesions: retrospective study of 124 cases. Acta Cytol. 2006;50(4):364–71.
5. Domanski HA, Akerman M, Engellau J, Gustafson P, Mertens F, Rydholm A. Fine-needle aspiration of neurilemoma (schwannoma). A clinicocytopathologic study of 116 patients. Diagn Cytopathol. 2006;34(6):403–12.
6. Wu JM, Sheth S, Ali SZ. Cytopathologic analysis of paraspinal masses: a study of 59 cases with clinicoradiologic correlation. Diagn Cytopathol. 2005;33(3):157–61.
7. Oliai BR, Sheth S, Burroughs FH, Ali SZ. "Parapharyngeal space" tumors: a cytopathological study of 24 cases on fine-needle aspiration. Diagn Cytopathol. 2005;32(1):11–5.
8. Laforga JB. Cellular schwannoma: report of a case diagnosed intraoperatively with the aid of cytologic imprints. Diagn Cytopathol. 2003;29(2):95–100.
9. Gupta RK, Cheung YK, Al Ansari AG, Naran S, Lallu S, Fauck R. Diagn Cytopathol. Diagnostic value of image-guided needle aspiration cytology in the assessment of vertebral and intervertebral lesions. 2002;27(4):191–6.
10. Klijanienko J, Caillaud JM, Lagacé R, Vielh P. Cytohistologic correlations of 24 malignant peripheral nerve sheath tumor (MPNST) in 17 patients: the Institut Curie experience. Diagn Cytopathol. 2002;27(2):103–8.
11. Kanahara T, Hirokawa M, Shimizu M, Terayama K, Nakamura E, Hino Y, Mikawa Y, Manabe T. Solitary fibrous tumor of the spinal cord. Report of a case with scrape cytology. Acta Cytol. 1999;43(3): 425–8.

Index

C.T. Welsh (ed.), *Intra-Operative Neuropathology for the Non-Neuropathologist: A Case-Based Approach*,
DOI 10.1007/978-1-4419-1167-4, © Springer Science+Business Media, LLC 2012